Essentials of Physical Medicine and Rehabilitation

Essentials of Physical Medicine and Rehabilitation

Zayne Oliver

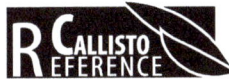

R CALLISTO REFERENCE

www.callistoreference.com

Callisto Reference,
118-35 Queens Blvd., Suite 400,
Forest Hills, NY 11375, USA

Visit us on the World Wide Web at:
www.callistoreference.com

ISBN: 978-1-64116-633-1 (Hardback)

Cataloging-in-Publication Data

Essentials of physical medicine and rehabilitation / Zayne Oliver.
   p. cm.
Includes bibliographical references and index.
ISBN 978-1-64116-633-1
1. Medicine, Physical. 2. Medical rehabilitation. 3. Medicine. 4. Rehabilitation. I. Oliver, Zayne.
RM700 .E77 2022
615.82--dc23

Table of Contents

Preface   **VII**

Chapter 1   Physical Medicine and Rehabilitation   1

• Physical Therapy   4
• Rehabilitation   9
• Areas of Physiotherapy   10
• Musculoskeletal Medicine   12

Chapter 2   Types of Physical Therapy and Rehabilitation   14

• Chest Physical Therapy   14
• Orthopedic Physical Therapy   17
• Geriatric Physical Therapy   19
• Neurological Physical Therapy   21
• Aquatic Therapy   23
• Cognitive Rehabilitation Therapy   32
• Cardiac Rehabilitation   35
• Robotic Neurorehabilitation   37

Chapter 3   Neuromuscular Medicine   41

• Neuromuscular Disorders   41
• Neuromuscular Medicine   60
• Neuromuscular Diseases and Rehabilitation   70
• Myotonic Dystrophy   97

Chapter 4   Pediatric Rehabilitation Medicine   104

• Pediatric Neuromuscular Disorders   104
• Cerebral Palsy   105
• Pediatric Muscular Dystrophies   112
• Pediatric Rehabilitation Medicine   125
• Pediatric Neurorehabilitation Medicine   126
• Pediatric Physical Therapy   138

Chapter 5   Role of Physical Medicine and Rehabilitation in Various Disorders   144
- Shoulder Disorders   144
- Low Back Pain   163
- Knee Injury   170
- Parkinson's Disease   176

Chapter 6   Rehabilitation of Sport-related Injuries   179
- Common Sports Injuries   179
- Sports Specific Rehabilitation   182
- Ankle and Foot Injuries in Athletes   194
- Sports Concussion   205
- Sports and Occupational Injuries to the Wrist and Hand   211
- Shin-Splint Syndrome   220
- Rehabilitation of the Overhead Athlete's Elbow   229

Permissions

Index

Preface

The branch of medicine which seeks to enhance and restore functional ability to the people suffering from physical impairments is known as physical medicine and rehabilitation. This field deals specifically with restoring optimal function to people with injuries to the nervous system, muscles, bones or ligaments. The major concern of this field is to enable the person to function optimally within the limitations placed upon them. These limitations can be caused by a disabling impairment or a disease process for which there is no known cure. There are various subspecialties within this discipline such as neuromuscular medicine, pain medicine, pediatric rehabilitation medicine and sports medicine. The topics covered in this extensive book deal with the core aspects of physical medicine and rehabilitation. It is an upcoming field of medicine that has undergone rapid development over the past few decades. This book includes contributions of experts which will provide innovative insights into this field.

To facilitate a deeper understanding of the contents of this book a short introduction of every chapter is written below:

Chapter 1- The branch of medicine that targets to improve and restore biomechanical movements, and functional ability and quality, of the human body is referred to as physical medicine and rehabilitation. It deals with the injuries related to the CNS, bones, muscles, tendons, etc. This chapter has been carefully written to provide an extensive understanding of physical medicine and rehabilitation.

Chapter 2- Physical therapy deals with the improvement of patient's health by the means of physical examination, diagnosis, prognosis and physical rehabilitation. It includes methodologies such as chest physical therapy, orthopedic physical therapy, geriatric physical therapy, cognitive rehabilitation therapy, robotic neurorehabilitation, etc. This chapter discusses these types of physical therapy and rehabilitation medicine in detail.

Chapter 3- Neuromuscular medicine is the product of amalgamation of neurology and physiatry which plays a vital role in the treatment of neuromuscular diseases. Some of the important areas covered in this field are neuromuscular diseases and rehabilitation, myotonic dystrophy, etc. The topics elaborated in this chapter will help in gaining a better perspective about neuromuscular medicine.

Chapter 4- The field of medicine which aims to prevent, detect, treat and manage congenital and childhood-onset physical disabilities is referred to as pediatric rehabilitation medicine. It includes pediatric muscular dystrophies, pediatric neurorehabilitation medicine, rehabilitation management, etc. All these diverse aspects of pediatric rehabilitation medicine have been carefully analyzed in this chapter.

Chapter 5- Physical medicine and rehabilitation has a wide domain which comprises of treatments for shoulder disorders, low back pain, knee injury, spinal cord injuries, Parkinson's disease, hemophilia, +-Guillain-Barre syndrome, etc. This chapter has been carefully written to provide an easy understanding of the aspects related to physical medicine and rehabilitation of various disorders.

Chapter 6- Physical medicine and rehabilitation play an important role in the area of sports nutrition. This chapter delves into rehabilitation of ankle and foot injuries in athletes, sports concussion, shin-splint syndrome, overhead athlete's elbow, hip and groin pain, hamstring injury, etc. to provide an extensive understanding of the subject.

Finally, I would like to thank the entire team involved in the inception of this book for their valuable time and contribution. This book would not have been possible without their efforts. I would also like to thank my friends and family for their constant support.

Zayne Oliver

Chapter 1

Physical Medicine and Rehabilitation

The branch of medicine that targets to improve and restore biomechanical movements, and functional ability and quality, of the human body is referred to as physical medicine and rehabilitation. It deals with the injuries related to the CNS, bones, muscles, tendons, etc. This chapter has been carefully written to provide an extensive understanding of physical medicine and rehabilitation.

Physical medicine and rehabilitation (PM&R), or physiatry, is a medical specialty focused on prevention, diagnosis, rehabilitation, and therapy for patients who experience functional limitations resulting from injury, disease, or malformation. Although the specialty is a relatively young one (with beginnings in the early twentieth century), fundamentals of the field originated during ancient times. The history of PM&R crosses many cultures and geographic boundaries.

Rehabilitation therapy, an essential component of the PM&R treatment approach, has a long history. Thousands of years ago the ancient Chinese employed Cong Fu, a movement therapy, to relieve pain; the Greek physician Herodicus described an elaborate system of gymnastic exercises for the prevention and treatment of disease in the fifth century BCE; and the Roman physician Galen described interventions to rehabilitate military injuries in the second century CE. During the Middle Ages, the philosopher-physician Maimonides emphasized Talmudic principles of healthy exercise habits, as well as diet, as preventive medicine in Medical Aphorisms, published between 1187-1190; and in 1569 the philologist-physician Mercurialis promoted gymnastics as both a preventive and a rehabilitative method in The Art of Gymnastics. In the eighteenth century, Niels Stenson explored the biomechanics of human motion and Joseph Clement Tissot's 1780 Medical and Surgical Gymnastics promoted the value of movement as an alternative to bed rest for patients recovering from surgery, facing neurological conditions, and recuperating after strokes. In the nineteenth century, the concept of neuromuscular re-education was proposed by Fulgence Raymond.

Physical Medicine Rehabilitation Today

Today, the Board of Physical Medicine and Rehabilitation defines physiatrists as:

"Nerve, muscle, and bone experts who treat injuries or illnesses that affect how you move diagnose and treat pain, restore maximum function lost through injury, illness or disabling conditions, treat the whole person, not just the problem area, lead a team of medical professionals, provide non-surgical treatments, [and] explain your medical problems and treatment/prevention plan".

As a general rule, many medical specialties focus on the acute management and stabilization of pathologic conditions (e.g., pneumonia or a fractured femur); PM&R also focuses on holistic patient-centered care that addresses social circumstances (e.g., type of job, hobbies), living space (e.g., number of steps to get into the house, presence of grab bars in the bathroom), and activities of daily living (e.g., proficiency in walking, washing, dressing, cooking, driving). Physiatrists customize treatment plans for patients based on these parameters. The physiatry treatment armamentarium often includes medications, therapeutic exercise, injections, physical modalities, and education.

By emphasizing prevention, diagnosis, and treatment of patients' functional limitations resulting from many different medical conditions, PM&R helps to maintain and restore optimal function for patients in many spheres of life including the social, emotional, medical, and vocational. Known as the quality-of-life medical specialty, PM&R aims to enhance a person's functional prognosis through a dynamic team-oriented approach. The physiatrist leads a multidisciplinary team that includes practitioners from physical therapy, occupational therapy, nursing, speech and language pathology, and other specialties. As team leaders, physiatrists champion the rights and autonomy of their patients by maximizing function and optimizing their living situations so that they can contribute to the community in the least restrictive setting. Physiatry's overarching commitment to optimizing the quality of life and neuromuscular function of an aging society has been recognized internationally.

Ethics in Physical Medicine and Rehabilitation

With the historical growth and evolution of the field of PM&R summarized above, a variety of ethical and moral issues has emerged. Kirschner identified general subsets of ethical issues confronted by physiatrists in contemporary practice and categorized their frequency: 24 percent involved health care reimbursement changes; 17 percent involved conflict among patients, physicians, interdisciplinary team members, and families around goal setting; and 7 percent involved assessing patients' decision-making capacity.

- Scarce resource allocation and the potential for discrimination against disabled people.

- The ethics of accommodating people with disability and chronic neuromuscular disorders, including in medical settings.

- Identifying optimally inclusive nomenclature and terminology (e.g., "physical diversity" rather than "disability").

- Conflict between the goals of promoting acceptance and accommodation for persons with disability on one hand and securing resources for restoration of functional efficiency and meaningful mission on the other hand.

- The ethics of rehabilitating persons with neurological and behavioural disorders with nosognosia (deficits of awareness), in which maximizing rehabilitation may mean abandoning or overriding patient autonomy.

Medical ethics provides a set of moral principles that guide the everyday practice of medicine. Jonsen propose that clinical problems be analyzed in light of four priorities or topics: medical indications, patient preferences (according to the principle of respect for autonomy, assessment of patients' expected quality of life, and context, such as economic constraints, procedures, and laws.

As team leaders, physiatrists must carefully and judiciously consider each of the above elements when making a decision. Additionally, consultation with the hospital medical ethics committee may be necessary. It may be challenging to reach consensus about a patient's treatment plan because health care clinicians consistently rate the quality of life of patients with disability or chronic illness lower than the patients rate it themselves, fostering disagreement between patient and treatment team.

Lewin define patient-centered care as care that shares decisions and interventions with the patient and views the patient as a whole person with social roles, rather than as an impaired organ. The role and ultimate obligation of the physiatrist as the leader of the interdisciplinary team is to thoroughly know and understand the patient as a person—including his or her interactions with family, employment, community, and environment. The physiatrist must have sufficient knowledge and experience to predict functional outcomes following rehabilitation for each patient. Sufficient evaluation must be carried out to confirm the diagnosis and prognosis. Optimal communication with the patient, family, and interdisciplinary team must take place throughout the patient's care.

Recently, an analysis model, PCEAM-R—Patient Centered Care Ethics Analysis Model for Rehabilitation—has been developed to guide ethical rehabilitative care, given the complexity of the care team, patient disablement, and a variety of possible interventions. This six-step process for ethical decision making is theoretically grounded in the International Classification of Functioning Disability and Health and has a sufficiently detailed list of questions to provide a comprehensive and balanced assessment of each patient's situation. Responsible physiatrists may want to consider using such guides to ensure high-quality care.

On an ongoing basis it is also the responsibility of the physiatrist as a citizen to support policies and laws that promote the independence and maximize the function of people with disabilities in the community.

Physical Therapy

Physical therapy (PT) is care that aims to ease pain and help you function, move, and live better. Physical therapists can help people who are having trouble moving after an injury or surgery. They also help people with conditions such as:

- Arthritis,

- Back or shoulder pain,

- Cerebral palsy,

- Osteoporosis (weak bones),

- Spinal cord injury,

- Stroke.

Physical therapists can help people gain strength and get moving again. They can help reduce or prevent pain and disability. Physical therapists provide care in hospitals, private practices, nursing homes, schools, rehabilitation centers, or in your home.

They use a variety of treatments, with a focus on physical activity and exercise. Goals include:

- Strengthening muscles that are weak from lack of use,

- Helping stiff joints move again,

- Helping you use your muscles correctly, so you can move with less pain and avoid injury.

But some physical therapy treatments are not useful. They can make your symptoms last longer, and even cause new problems.

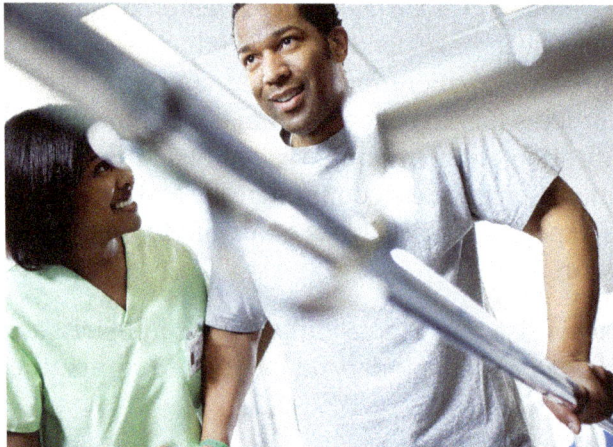

Avoid Treatments that won't Help

Most insurance plans pay for a limited number of physical therapy visits. If your treatment doesn't help, then you have wasted those visits.

Also, if treatment doesn't help, people are more likely to seek unnecessary tests, injections, and surgery. These can be costly and risky.

They can lead to harm and to more tests and treatments. And your costs go up. Here's why:

Heat Treatments

The problem: Treatments include hot packs and deep heat machines, such as ultrasound. They can feel good on a painful back, shoulder, or knee. They may help relax you before exercise, but there is no proof that they have any lasting effect.

For example: Studies have found that deep-heat ultrasound, added to an exercise program, does not improve arthritis of the knee. It's better to learn specific exercises and new ways to do things.

The harms: Many people are afraid to be physically active when they're in pain. Physical therapists may support these fears by using heat treatments. But avoiding movement only makes the problem worse. This can lead to unnecessary medical procedures, such as knee surgery or steroid injections for back pain.

When to Consider Heat

- Home heat treatments, such as a hot bath or shower or a heating pad, can help give temporary relief of aches and pains.

- Calcific tendonitis is a painful shoulder condition. Deep heat using ultrasound can help.

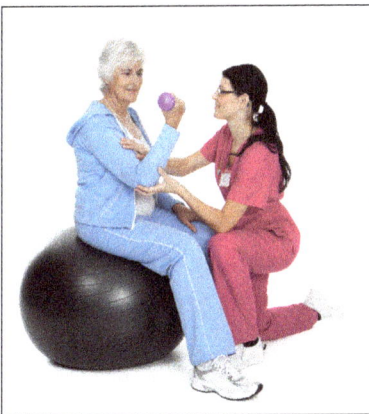

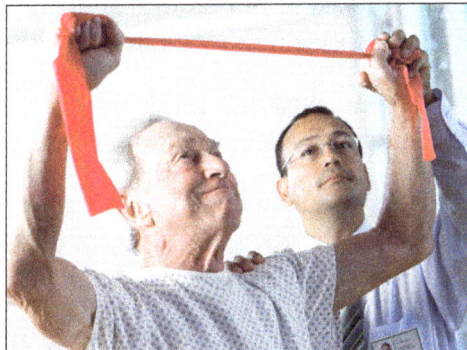

The Wrong Kind of Strength Training for Older Adults

The problem: Many older adults have weak muscles—due to lack of activity, hospitalization, or surgery. This can cause problems with walking, balance, rising from a chair, and other everyday activities. The risk of falls increases.

The right strength training program can make you stronger and help prevent falls. A physical therapist can teach you how to use exercise machines, free weights, elastic bands, or your own body to build strength. But the exercises may be too easy. The therapist may be afraid that you'll be hurt.

Studies show that a challenging program offers the most benefits, even for seniors in nursing homes. The therapist should match the program to your abilities. When you can do an exercise easily, the therapist should add weight, repetitions, or new exercises.

The harms: If strength training isn't challenging, it is a waste of time and money. You will still have problems from weak muscles. And you will still be at risk of falling.

When to Go Easy on Muscles

- Start out with lighter weights so you can learn the correct way to use them.

- Don't do strength training if you have a painful, inflamed joint, such as a swollen elbow or knee.

Bed Rest for Blood Clots

The problem: Older adults and people who have had surgery have a risk of deep vein thrombosis (DVT). This is a blood clot in a deep vein—usually in the leg.

The main treatment for DVT is medicine that dissolves blood clots. In addition, patients are often put on bed rest.

The purpose of bed rest is to keep the clot from breaking loose. A loose clot may travel to the lungs and block blood flow in the lungs. This is called a pulmonary embolism (PE), and it can be fatal. But studies show that bed rest doesn't help. People who walk around with a clot are no more likely to develop a PE than people who lie in bed.

Also, getting up and walking has many benefits. It makes people feel better. It relieves pain and swelling in the leg. And it reduces the risk of more leg problems.

A physical therapist can help you start walking as soon as the clot-preventing medicine starts working. Or the therapist or your doctor can tell you how active to be on your own.

The harms: Bed rest can make a clot larger and lead to new clots. And you will have a higher risk of complications, such as pneumonia. Your entire body will become weaker.

When to Consider Bed Rest for DVT

You may need bed rest if:

- You can't take clot-preventing medicines.

- You have another medical reason for bed rest such as bleeding in the brain from a stroke, or severe breathing problems.

Exercise Machines (CPM) after Total Knee Replacement

The problem: Most people start physical therapy within 24 hours after knee replacement surgery. The therapist should show you how to exercise your knee, walk, and get in and out of a bed or chair. This helps you move your knee again. It reduces the risk of a blood clot in the leg and shortens hospital stays.

But some surgeons recommend that you also use a continuous passive motion (CPM) machine. A CPM machine keeps moving the knee for several hours a day while you're in bed. A physical therapist teaches you how to use the machine.

But studies show that adding a CPM machine to physical therapy doesn't improve pain. It doesn't help you bend or straighten your knee better. And it doesn't help you return to normal activities or improve your quality of life.

In fact, people do just as well with physical therapy whether they add a CPM machine or not.

The harms: CPM is a large, heavy machine. It is hard to put on. You have to pay to rent it. And you may stay in bed longer, instead of getting up and being active.

When to Consider CPM

CPM may be helpful if:

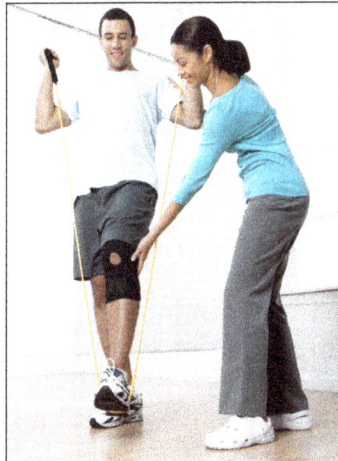

- You had a serious complication from the surgery, such as a stroke or respiratory failure. In this case you may need more bed rest.

- You are recovering from a second knee replacement operation because the first one failed.

Whirlpools for Wound Care

The problem: Physical therapists are often asked to treat wounds that are slow to heal, chronic, or infected. One treatment uses a whirlpool bath to soak and clean the wound. But there is little evidence that whirlpools help. And they can cause infections.

There are safer, gentler, more effective ways to clean wounds. The therapist can:

- Rinse the wound with a saltwater wash.

- Spray liquid on areas of the wound with a single-use sterile device.

The Harms

- If the tub is not clean, bacteria can spread from person to person.

- Bacteria can spread from other parts of your own body to the wound.

- An infected wound heals more slowly and you may need antibiotics.

- If your immune system is weak, the infection can spread to the blood and cause a serious condition called sepsis.

- Chemicals used to clean the tub and disinfect the water can damage the new skin cells on the wound.

- Whirlpool jets can harm fragile new tissue growing in the wound.

- Long soaking can break down skin around the wound.

- The placement of the leg can cause swelling. People who have vein problems may have serious complications.

When to Consider Whirlpool Therapy

Never use whirlpool therapy to treat open wounds. It may help sports injuries such as strained muscles, but the benefit has not been proven.

Rehabilitation

Rehabilitation medicine focuses on rehabilitating patients with physical disabilities caused by injuries or diseases. Also known as physical medicine and rehabilitation or physiatry, this branch of medicine is dedicated to helping patients reach their full potential despite their physical limitations.

A specialist who practices in this field is called a physiatrist, not to be confused with a psychiatrist, who focuses on mental health. However, in some cases, both medical professionals work closely together to achieve a common goal.

People with physical disabilities find it difficult to live a normal, productive life. It was with this concern that physiatry was established. Unlike the majority of other branches of medicine, physiatry's primary objective is not to diagnose or treat certain conditions but to help patients overcome the limitations that their disabilities impose. As such, physiatrists are trained in the rehabilitation of a wide variety of conditions, such as spinal cord injuries and other conditions that result in a physical disability.

Anybody of any age with a disability that affects their way of life and those who have incurable diseases that create functional problems are eligible for rehabilitation medicine.

Some of the most common conditions that require rehabilitation medicine include osteoporosis, chronic back pain, spinal cord injuries, osteoarthritis, ankylosing spondylitis, and fibromyalgia. Physiatrists also provide treatment for sports-related injuries and musculoskeletal problems.

In terms of expectations, the results of treatment differ from patient to patient. Some respond better to treatment than others while some may need more time before any significant improvements to their condition can be noted. However, with continuous treatment and a significant amount of effort, a patient's condition should improve immensely.

How does the Procedure Work?

The exact treatment procedures differ based on the type of treatment and the condition being treated. However, prior to receiving any form of treatment, physiatrists typically perform a thorough physical examination and conduct imaging tests so they are able to formulate a targeted rehabilitation plan.

When diagnosing the patient's condition, physiatrists rely on a number of diagnostic tools that focus on identifying nerve or muscle damage. These include electromyography (EMG), a tool that evaluates the electrical activity produced by different muscles, and nerve conduction studies (NCS), which evaluate the condition of the nerves while in a relaxed or stimulated situation.

In addition to the above procedures, a physiatrist may also opt to use other tools, such as ultrasound, nerve stimulators, muscle and nerve biopsy and prosthetics, among many others.

Possible Risks and Complications

Although rehabilitation medicine programs are based on the patient's condition and exact need, they still carry some degree of risk and possible complications.

For instance, patients who attempt to perform certain exercises or movements in order to build muscles and regain some functions are at risk of injuries. Also, it is common for patients with incurable diseases to develop complications, which is why physiatrists work closely with the attending physician so that any complications can be prevented or managed in a timely manner.

The majority of treatment methods used in rehabilitation medicine are non-surgical. As much as possible, physiatrists use conservative treatment methods to lower the risks of complications. However, if non-surgical methods fail to improve a patient's condition, surgery may be considered. If so, another set of risks and possibilities of complications will arise because of the surgical procedure.

Risks and complications are not limited to the physical aspect of a patient's condition. In fact, patients with disabilities have psychological problems that also need to be addressed during treatment. Many of them go through an emotional rollercoaster when undergoing rehabilitation. Therefore, the patient's emotional state of mind is also closely monitored during treatment to prevent the patient from going into an emotional state that will reduce the effectiveness of the treatment.

Areas of Physiotherapy

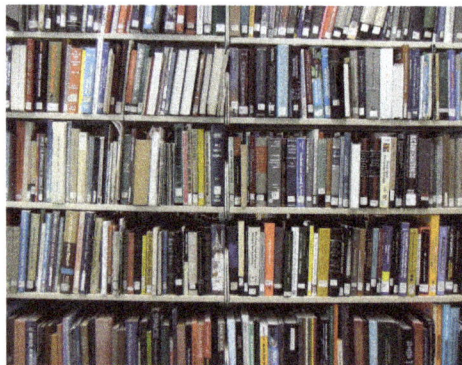

Physiotherapy is an extremely wide field of study. It can be classified into different areas of focus, patient age groups, gender and type of activities (or sub-specialties). As a result, people often get confused about what it is, who it is for and what it does. Most often one gets to learn about physiotherapy you come into contact with it for your own health matters or know someone close who is undergoing treatment.

Broadly, physiotherapy can be segregated into 3 main areas – Musculoskeletal, Cardio-Respiratory (sometimes also referred to Cardio-Pulmonary) and Neurology.

- Musculoskeletal: This is the area that deals with injuries related to the muscles, bones and joints of the human muscle and skeletal system. Conditions such as back pain, tennis elbows and ankle sprains fall into this category. Private clinics outside of the hospital setting typically focus on this area. This area is sometimes referred to as Orthopaedics.

- Cardio-Respiratory: This area deals with conditions related to the lung and circulatory system (e.g. heart). Conditions such as fall into this category are bronchial asthma, chronic obstructive lungs disease and pneumothorax. Generally, this is an in-patient area. Meaning patient are still warded in the hospital such as after cardiac surgery. Out-patient care such as chest percussion treatment is sometimes called upon for patient who suffers from attacks of chest congestion and find it difficult to breath.

- Neurology: This area deals with rehabilitation of patients recovering from neurological condition such as stroke, cerebral palsy. Stroke depending on its severity often lead to partial paralysis of some part of the body. Neuro-physiotherapy helps the patient to recover some of the mobility and control of these body parts. This is often confused with the Musculoskeletal area of physiotherapy as it includes improving muscle strength and control. The key difference here is the source of the muscular dysfunction.

Patient Demographics

Each of these areas can be further broken down into three broad age classification: Pediatrics, adult and geriatrics.

Pediatrics deals with young infants and children. Teenagers typically are classified as adult though these age group do have specific needs that needs to be managed separately such growth spurts in the bone structures.

Adults are the largest group of patients for physiotherapy as they represent the bulk of the population. However, with a rapidly aging population, geriatric physiotherapy for older adults is increasingly playing a larger role in the community.

Gender Classification

Men and women sometimes have different requirements when treating certain conditions dues to the difference to their physiology. Some are clearly visible such as the bone structure. One example is women having wider hips than men. This difference plays an importance role in the treatment of knee pains.

Other differences are not as visible such as hormonal difference such estrogen and its impact on bone density as women age.

Activities and Sub-specialties

With each area, there are further sub-specialties such as sports physiotherapy. Sports physiotherapy is a sub-specialty of the Musculoskeletal area. It can be further classified to the various patient demographics. Treating young children and teenagers the same as adult with sports physiotherapy can led to irreparable damage to their growth and subsequently adult musculoskeletal frame.

Another example of sub-specialty is women health and in particularly pregnant women and post-natal women.

Musculoskeletal Medicine

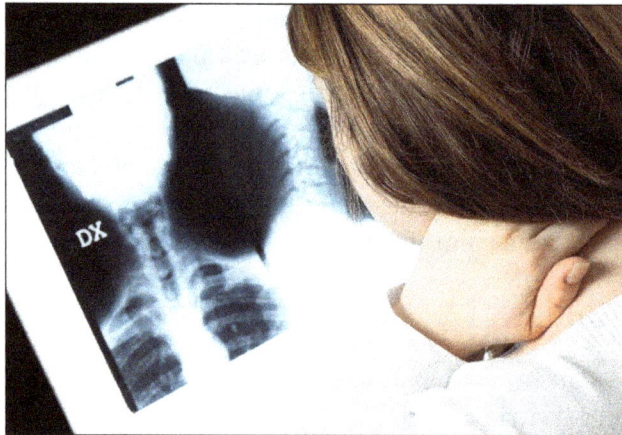

Musculoskeletal Medicine is a branch of medicine which specialises in the diagnosis and management of conditions affecting the musculoskeletal system (bones, muscles, joints, tendons and ligaments).

Problems diagnosed by Musculoskeletal Specialists include muscular and soft tissues injuries or disorders, bone disorders, joint injuries and arthritis of various kinds and simple or complex pain conditions that affect a person's movement patterns. These conditions become more common as a person gets older, and can also occur as a result of injuries.

Treatment by Musculoskeletal Medicine doctors includes: providing information about the condition, pain management strategies, manual therapy, trigger point treatment, soft tissue and peripheral and spinal joint injections, pain implants (including spinal cord stimulation), advise on medication, advise regarding exercise and rehabilitation programmes and appropriate referrals, if required.

Musculoskeletal Medicine doctors work closely with your GP as well as health practitioners in other disciplines to ensure your medical needs are met effectively and safely. These include physiotherapists, psychologists, surgeons, pain physicians, neurologists, psychiatrists, rehabilitation physicians and occupational physicians.

References

- History-physical-medicine-and-rehabilitation-and-its-ethical-dimensions: journalofethics.ama-assn.org, Retrieved 02 January, 2019

- Physical-Therapy-APTA, wp-content: choosingwisely.org, Retrieved 23 March, 2019

- Rehabilitation-medicine-physicians: docdoc.com.sg, Retrieved 19 May, 2019

- Areas-of-physiotherapy: coreconcepts.com.sg, Retrieved 03 July, 2019

- The-physiatric-history-and-physical-examination: clinicalgate.com, Retrieved 14 August, 2019

- Musculoskeletal-medicine, healthcare-services-pain-management-treatments: precisionhealth.com.au, Retrieved 25 January, 2019

Chapter 2

Types of Physical Therapy and Rehabilitation

Physical therapy deals with the improvement of patient's health by the means of physical examination, diagnosis, prognosis and physical rehabilitation. It includes methodologies such as chest physical therapy, orthopedic physical therapy, geriatric physical therapy, cognitive rehabilitation therapy, robotic neurorehabilitation, etc. This chapter discusses these types of physical therapy and rehabilitation medicine in detail.

Chest Physical Therapy

Chest physical therapy (CPT or Chest PT) is an airway clearance technique (ACT) to drain the lungs, and may include percussion (clapping), vibration, deep breathing, and huffing or coughing.

With chest physical therapy (CPT), the person gets in different positions to use gravity to drain mucus (postural drainage) from the five lobes of the lungs. Each position is designed so that a major part of the lung is facing downward. When combined with percussion, it may be known as postural drainage and percussion (PD&P). This is where a caregiver or partner can clap and or vibrate the person's chest to further dislodge and move the mucus to the larger airways where it can be coughed or huffed out of the body.

CPT is easy to do. For a child with cystic fibrosis, CPT can be done by anyone, including parents, siblings, and friends. It can also be done by physical therapists, respiratory therapists, or nurses during care center visits or in the hospital.

How to do it

With postural drainage, the person lies or sits in various positions so the part of the lung to be drained is as high as possible. That part of the lung is then drained using percussion, vibration, and gravity. Your care team may tailor these positions to your or your child's needs.

When the person with CF is in one of the positions, the caregiver can clap on the person's chest wall. This is usually done for three to five minutes and is sometimes followed by vibration over the same area for approximately 15 seconds (or during five exhalations). The person is then encouraged to cough or huff forcefully to get the mucus out of the lungs.

Clapping (percussion) by the caregiver on the chest wall over the part of the lung to be drained helps move the mucus into the larger airways. The hand is cupped as if to hold water but with the palm facing down. The cupped hand curves to the chest wall and traps a cushion of air to soften the clapping.

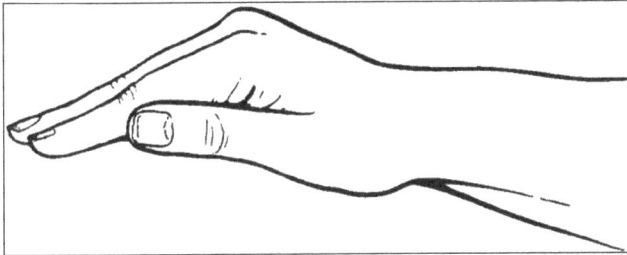

Percussion is done forcefully and with a steady beat. Each beat should have a hollow sound. Most of the movement is in the wrist with the arm relaxed, making percussion less tiring to do. If the hand is cupped properly, percussion should not be painful or sting.

Special attention must be taken to not clap over the:

- Spine,

- Breastbone,

- Stomach,

- Lower ribs or back (to prevent injury to the spleen on the left, the liver on the right and the kidneys in the lower back).

Different devices may be used in place of the traditional cupped palm method for percussion. Ask your CF doctor or respiratory therapist to recommend one that may work best for you.

Vibration is a technique that gently shakes the mucus so it can move into the larger airways. The caregiver places a firm hand on the chest wall over the part of the lung being drained and tenses the muscles of the arm and shoulder to create a fine shaking motion. Then, the caregiver applies a light pressure over the area being vibrated. (The caregiver may also place one hand over the other, then press the top and bottom hand into each other to vibrate).

Vibration is done with the flattened hand, not the cupped hand. Exhalation should be as slow and as complete as possible.

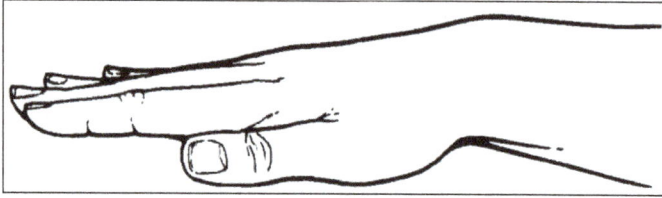

Deep breathing moves the loosened mucus and may lead to coughing. Breathing with the diaphragm (belly breathing or lower chest breathing) is used to help the person take deeper breaths and get the air into the lower lungs. The belly moves outward when the person breathes in and sinks in when he or she breathes out. Your CF respiratory or physical therapist can help you learn more about this type of breathing.

How Long does CPT Take?

Generally, each treatment session can last between 20 to 40 minutes. CPT is best done before meals or one-and-a-half to two hours after eating, to decrease the chance of vomiting. Early morning and bedtimes are usually recommended. The length of CPT and the number of times a day it is done may need to be increased if the person is more congested or getting sick. Your CF doctor or respiratory therapist can recommend what positions, how often and how long CPT should be done.

Doing CPT Comfortably and Carefully

Both the person with CF and the caregiver should be comfortable during CPT. Before starting, the person should remove tight clothing, jewellery, buttons, and zippers around the neck, chest and waist. Light, soft clothing, such as a T-shirt, may be worn. Do not do CPT on bare skin. The caregiver should remove rings and other bulky jewellery, such as watches or bracelets. Keep a supply of tissues or a place to cough out the mucus nearby.

The caregiver should not lean forward when doing percussion, but should remain in an upright position to protect his or her back. The surface that the person with CF lies on should be at a comfortable height for the caregiver.

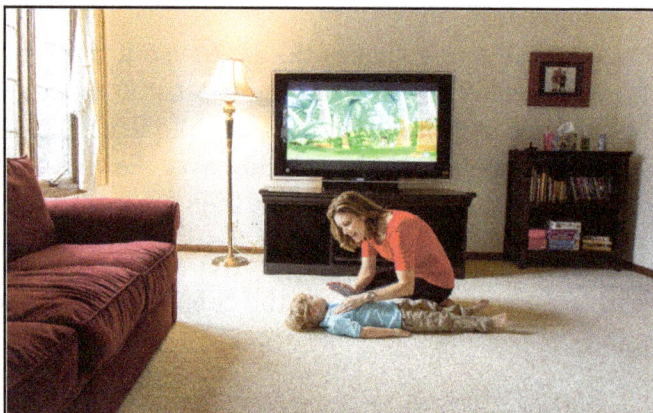

Many families find it helpful to use pillows, sofa cushions, or bundles of newspapers under pillows for support, as well as cribs with adjustable mattress heights/tilts, foam wedges, or bean bag chairs while doing CPT. Infants can be positioned with or without pillows in the caregiver's lap.

Purchasing Equipment

Equipment such as drainage tables, electrical and nonelectrical palm percussors, and vibrators may be helpful. These can be purchased from medical equipment stores. Older children and adults may find percussors useful when doing their own CPT. Talk to your doctor or respiratory therapist at your CF care center about equipment for CPT.

Orthopedic Physical Therapy

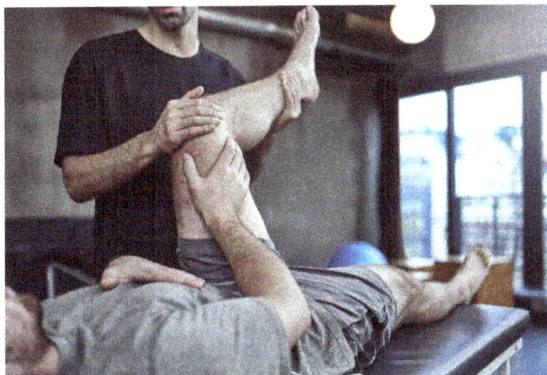

If you have an injury or illness that affects your bones, joints, muscles, tendons, or ligaments, you may benefit from the skilled services of a physical therapist trained in orthopedic physical therapy.

These days, medical professionals are ultra-specialized, and physical therapists are no exception to this trend. Some physical therapists specialize in helping patients who have orthopedic conditions—those injuries that cause impairments or dysfunction to various bony and soft tissue structures of the body.

Conditions in Orthopedic Physical Therapy

Orthopedic physical therapy focuses on treating conditions affecting the musculoskeletal system, which is made up of your joints, muscles, bones, ligaments, and tendons. Orthopedic injuries and conditions may include:

- Fractures,
- Muscle strains,

- Ligament sprains,

- Post-operative conditions,

- Tendonitis,

- Bursitis.

An injury to a bone, joint, tendon, ligament, or muscle may cause pain, limited functional mobility, and loss of strength or range of motion. These impairments may prevent you from enjoying your normal work or recreational activities. The focus of orthopedic physical therapy is to help your injury heal properly and improve your strength, range of motion, and overall functional mobility.

After surgery, you may have specific limitations that your surgeon wants you to adhere to. Your orthopedic physical therapist can help guide you through your post-operative rehab program to get you back to your normal lifestyle quickly and safely.

Any condition that causes pain or limited functional mobility as a result of an injury to bony or soft tissue structures in your body may benefit from the skilled services of orthopedic physical therapy.

Tools of the Trade

Your orthopedic physical therapist uses specific tools to help you during your rehab. These may include:

- Therapeutic modalities like heat, ice, ultrasound, or electrical stimulation,

- Assistive devices, such as walkers or canes,

- Orthotics and prosthetics,

- Exercise tools and equipment,

- Evaluation and assessment tools,

- Mobilization or soft tissue massages instruments.

While your PT may use various instruments and tools to help you move better and get better, exercise is often your main tool to help you recover fully and prevent future orthopedic problems. Exercises in orthopedic physical therapy often involve:

- Strengthening exercises,

- Stretching and flexibility exercises,

- Exercises to improve range of motion,

- Balance exercises,

- Functional mobility exercises,

- Endurance exercises,

- Plyometric and jumping-type exercises.

Geriatric Physical Therapy

Geriatric physical therapy was defined as a medical specialty in 1989 and covers a broad area of concerns regarding people as they continue the process of aging, although it commonly focuses on older adults.

Geriatric physical therapy covers a wide area of issues concerning people as they go through normal adult aging but is usually focused on the older adult. There are many conditions that affect many people as they grow older and include but are not limited to the following: arthritis, osteoporosis, cancer, Alzheimer's disease, hip and joint replacement, balance disorders, incontinence, etc. Geriatric physical therapists specialize in providing therapy for such conditions in older adults.

Among the conditions that may be treated through the use of geriatric physical therapy are osteoporosis, arthritis, alzheimer's disease, cancer, joint replacement, hip replacement, and more. The form of therapy is used in order to restore mobility, increase fitness levels, reduce pain, and to provide additional benefits.

Geriatric physical therapy is a proven means for older adults from every level of physical ability to improve their balance and strength, build their confidence, and remain active. A number of people are familiar with physical therapy as a form of treatment to pursue after an accident, or in relation to a condition such as a stroke. Physical therapy is useful for many additional reasons, such as improving balance, strength, mobility, and overall fitness. All of these are factors which older adults may benefit from, contributing to their physical abilities and helping to maintain their independence for longer periods of time. Physical therapy can also help older adults to avoid falls, something that is crucial to this population.

Falling is one of the greatest risks older adults face, often leading to things such as hip fractures which then lead to a downward health spiral. In fact, falling is such an issue among older adults that the Center for Disease Control and Prevention has reported that one-third of all people over the age of sixty-five fall every year, making falls the leading cause of injury among people from this age group. Hundreds of thousands of older adults experience falls and resulting hip fractures every year, with resulting hospitalizations. Most of the people who experience a hip fracture stay in the hospital for a minimum of one week, with approximately twenty-percent dying within a year due to the injury. Unfortunately, a number of the remaining eighty-percent do not return to their previous level of functioning. Physical therapy can help older adults to remain both strong and independent, as well as productive.

Forms of Geriatric Physical Therapy

Exercise: Exercise is defined as any form of physical activity that is beyond what the person does while performing their daily tasks. Exercise is something that is designed to both maintain and improve a person's coordination, muscle strength, flexibility and physical endurance, as well as their balance. It is meant to increase their mobility and lessen their chance of injury through falling. Exercise in relation to geriatric therapy might include activities such as stretching, walking, weight lifting, aquatic therapy, and specific exercises that are geared towards a particular injury or limitation. A physical therapist works with the person, teaching them to exercise on their own, so they may continue their exercise program at home.

Manual Therapy: Manual therapy is applied with the goals of improving the person's circulation and restoring mobility they may have lost due to an injury or lack of use. This form of therapy is also used to reduce pain. Manual therapy can include manipulation of the person's joints and muscles, as well as massage.

Education: Education is important to the success and effectiveness of geriatric physical therapy. People are taught ways of performing daily tasks safely. Physical therapists also teach people how to use assistive devices, as well as how to protect themselves from further injury. Older adults can utilize physical therapy as a means for regaining their independence. Physical therapy can help seniors to feel better, as well as to enjoy a higher quality of life.

Physical Therapists

Physical therapists provide people with a variety of services. They work with people individually, evaluating their physical capabilities and designing specific programs of exercise, education and wellness for them. Physical therapists also work with other health care providers to coordinate the person's care.

Physical therapists must have completed their coursework in the biological, medical, psychological and physical sciences. They must have graduated from an accredited education program, and have completed a bachelors, masters, or doctoral degree with specialty clinical experience in physical therapy. Many physical therapists choose to seek additional expertise in clinical specialties, although every physical therapist must meet licensure requirements in their state.

The potential for age-related bodily changes to be misunderstood can lead to limitations of daily activities. The usual process of aging does not need to result in pain, or decreased physical mobility. A physical therapist can be a source of information for understanding changes in the body, they can offer assistance for regaining lost abilities, or for development of new ones. A physical therapist can work with older adults to help them understand the physiological and anatomical changes that occur with the aging process.

Physical therapists evaluate and develop specifically designed, therapeutic exercise programs. Physical therapy intervention can prevent life-long disability, restoring the person's level of functioning to its highest level. A physical therapist uses things such as treatments with modalities, exercises, educational information, and screening programs to accomplish a number of goals with the person they are working with, such as:

- Reduce pain.

- Improve sensation, joint proprioception.

- Increase overall fitness through exercise programs.

- Suggest assistive devices to promote independence.

- Recommend adaptations to make the person's home accessible and safe.

- Prevent further decline in functional abilities through education, energy conservation techniques, joint protection.

- Increase, restore or maintain range of motion, physical strength, flexibility, coordination, balance and endurance.

- Teach positioning, transfers, and walking skills to promote maximum function and independence within the person's capability.

There are various common conditions that can be effectively treated through physical therapy. Among the specific diseases and conditions that might affect older adults which can be improved with physical therapy are arthritis, osteoarthritis, stroke, Parkinson's disease, cancer, amputations, urinary and fecal incontinence, and cardiac and pulmonary diseases. Conditions such as Alzheimer's disease, dementia's, coordination and balance disorders, joint replacements, hip fractures, functional limitations related to mobility, orthopedic or sports injuries can also be improved through geriatric physical therapy.

Neurological Physical Therapy

Neurological Physical Therapy encompasses specialized comprehensive evaluation and treatment of individuals with movement problems due to disease or injury of the nervous system. Advanced Physical Therapy provides individualized one on one treatment with primary focus on restoring function and improving overall quality of life.

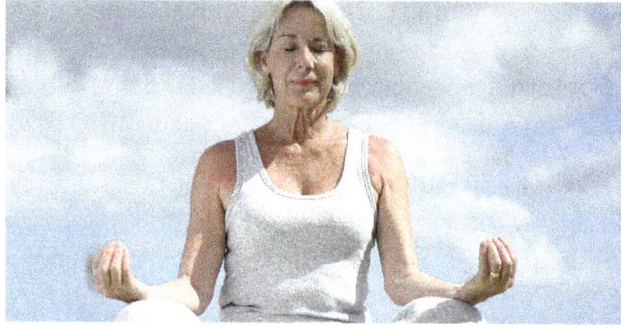

Commonly treated conditions include:

- Stroke,

- Traumatic brain injury,

- Spinal cord injury,

- Parkinson's Disease,

- Multiple Sclerosis,

- Guillain Barre Syndrome,

- Ataxia,

- Amyotrophic lateral sclerosis,

- Polyneuropathies,

- Progressive neurological conditions,

- Spasticity/tone.

Neurological physical therapy is extremely important for those patients who have had or who currently have neurological diseases or injuries. The brain and spinal cord and the central nervous system control movement and sensation. Injuries to these areas, the brain or spinal cord can cause death of the cells that control certain movements and sensations, and therefore people lose function. Without neurological physical therapy following a neurological injury, patients may lose many functions and not be able to perform certain activities. Decreased intensity of activity leads to many other health problems such as diabetes, heart problems, lung problems, decreased independence, and an overall poor quality of life.

Following the neurological disorder or injury, there is a certain amount of time when the cells that are not injured in the brain and spinal cord can learn to control the missing functions. Physical therapists are very well-informed about human movement and can teach patients how to move correctly again. This skilled assistance can help patients regain some to most of the functions they lost because of the injury. Most of the patients can learn to live their lives independently again, which makes them happier with their lives and contributes to their overall quality of life.

Neurological physical therapy treatment:

- Restore range of motion.
- Improve functional movement and strength.
- Gait Training.
- Postural re-alignment.
- Improve safety of transfers and mobility.
- Balance re-training and decrease risk of fall.
- Core stabilization.
- Activities of Daily Living (ADL) performance.
- Visual Perceptual Skill retraining.
- Cardiovascular endurance.
- Improve motor planning and motor control.
- Decrease spasticity/tone.
- Prosthesis/orthoses training.
- Equipment evaluation/recom,mendation to include wheelchairs, cane, walkers or crutches.

Aquatic Therapy

Aquatic therapy is physical therapy that takes place in a pool or other aquatic environment under the supervision of a trained healthcare professional. Aquatic therapy is also known as water therapy, aquatic rehabilitation, aqua therapy, pool therapy, therapeutic aquatic exercise or hydrotherapy.

Aquatic therapy is considered an add-on certification for physical therapists and athletic trainers who often work closely with occupational therapists and exercise physiologists to develop a plan of care for each client.

Common goals of aqua therapy programs include:

- Improving flexibility.

- Improving balance and coordination.

- Building muscle strength and endurance.

- Assisting with gait and locomotion.

- Reducing stress and promoting relaxation.

Aquatic therapy is different from aquatic exercise or aquatic fitness because it is a physical medicine and rehabilitation specialty that requires the involvement of a trained professional and is covered by many insurance providers due to the personalized nature of the treatment. Aquatic exercise does not need to be supervised by a trained professional. It is also not covered by insurance, and it often takes place in a group setting that includes multiple people with different levels of physical fitness.

Aquatic therapy should not be confused with adaptive aquatics, either. Adaptive aquatics is the process of teaching people with disabilities how to swim safely in the water. Aquatic therapy does not focus on teaching clients how to swim.

Water therapy services are generally offered in hospitals, sports medicine clinics and traditional outpatient rehabilitation centers. Senior living centers may also provide aquatic therapy services as a way to encourage their residents to maintain or improve fitness levels, balance and strength.

Water therapy has been used for thousands of years throughout the world. Consider the following examples:

- Ancient Greeks and Romans bathed in hot springs to improve circulation and promote relaxation.

- Hippocrates recommended bathing in spring water as a way to treat sickness.

- Swiss monks were known to use thermal waters to treat sick or disabled people in their community.

- Japanese hot springs, or onsens, are said to have medicinal effects that include healing chronic pain, treating skin problems, curing menstrual disorders and relieving constipation.

- German physicians were firm believers in pediatric water therapy. Water birthing was very popular throughout Germany in the 1960s and 1970s.

Conditions that can be Helped by Water Therapy

Water therapy may be helpful for clients suffering from the following conditions:

- Arthritis,

- Arthroscopic surgery recovery,

- Autism,

- Balance disorders,

- Bursitis,

- Cerebral palsy,

- Chronic pain,

- Depression,

- Idiopathic joint pain,

- Joint reconstruction surgery recovery,

- Joint replacement surgery recovery,

- Lower back pain,

- Osteoarthritis,

- Orthopedic injuries,

- Parkinson's disease,

- Multiple sclerosis,

- Rheumatoid arthritis,

- Scoliosis,

- Stress,

- Spinal cord injury,

- Sprains and strains,

- Stroke,

- Tendonitis,

- Traumatic Brain Injury.

People of all ages can enjoy water therapy benefits, including children with special needs and senior citizens. A trained therapist can create a session that takes into account any age-related physical limitations to promote a positive therapeutic experience.

Safety of Aquatic Exercise Programs

Even though aqua therapy typically takes place in a fairly shallow pool, it is not risk free. To provide a safe environment for clients, aquatic therapy practitioners should be trained in first aid, CPR, oxygen administration, automated external defibrillation, blood-borne pathogens and risk awareness (check local codes for actual requirements).

The suitability for aquatic therapy for a client should be decided on a case-by-case basis. Here are some situations where aqua therapy may not be an appropriate course of treatment:

- High fever.

- Open wounds (unless covered with bio-occlusive dressing).

- Incontinence.

- Uncontrolled seizure disorders.

- COPD or other similar respiratory issues.

- Currently taking medication that could alter cognition.

- Client is currently pregnant and experiencing complications.

- Chlorine or bromine allergy.

- Serious fear of water.

- Clients with Hepatitis A.

Helping Clients become Comfortable in the Water

Despite the many benefits of aqua therapy, some clients are hesitant to try this form of rehabilitation. For example, wearing a swimsuit in a public space can feel uncomfortable for clients.. Some clients may also physically struggle to dress properly for a therapy session. This requires the therapist to display compassion, empathy and understanding. There are many ways to address this self-image issue by offering alternatives such as shorts and a comfortable t-shirt for aquatic therapy, keeping dressing rooms and therapy pool separate from other therapy areas so that the session is semi-private and offering suits that are easier for those with arthritis or physical ailments.

When working with a client suffering from a visual impairment, it's recommended that the therapist orient that person to the pool before the session. The therapist should point out helpful landmarks, such as chairs and ladders, as they assist the client with walking around the perimeter of the therapy pool.

Ai Chi Aquatic Therapy Exercises

Ai Chi is a form of water therapy that was created in 1993 by Jun Konno, and it combines elements of Tai chi chuan and qigong to relax and strengthen the body. Exercises use diaphragmatic breathing and active progressive resistance training while integrating mental, physical and spiritual energy. It's a combination of both Eastern and Western beliefs.

Clients generally practice Ai Chi while they are standing in shoulder-depth water. The initial focus is on mastering deep breathing patterns, with clients then progressing into gentle movement of the upper and lower extremities. Throughout the process, careful attention is paid to body alignment and breathing to induce a calm, meditative state of mind.

It is hypothesized that Ai Chi can be useful in fall prevention programs for the elderly. Tai chi has long been used to improve balance in seniors, but Ai Chi provides an enhanced method of developing the lateral stability and stepping skills that play a crucial role in reducing fall risk.

Aqua Running

Also called deep-water running or aqua jogging, aqua running is a form of running in water that uses a flotation belt to support the head and upper body above water while preserving "normal" biomechanics. This type of aquatic therapy allows clients to experience the benefits of performing rehabilitation protocols without impact on joints.

Aqua running in deep water or on an underwater treadmill is most commonly used to help speed the recovery of injured athletes or to improve the fitness of people who require a low-impact aerobic workout.

For overweight or obese people who are physically unable to run on dry land, aqua jogging is a very effective weight loss technique. Since water is denser than air, aqua jogging burns more calories per minute than running on dry land. The pressure of the water also helps to allow the same intensity of exercise at a lower heart rate.

Aside from its use as a therapeutic technique, aqua running has a history of being a popular competitive sport. The Aqua Jogging World Championships are held each year in Finland and attract a large number of skilled athletes.

Bad Ragaz Ring Method for Water Therapy Exercises

The Bad Ragaz Ring Method for aqua therapy was developed by a team of physiotherapists in Bad Ragaz, Switzerland. The goal was to develop a water-based strengthening and mobilizing resistive exercise model. Their work combines elements of aquatic exercise techniques developed in the 1930s by German physician Knupfer with the 1950s and 1960s research of American neurophysiologist Herman Kabat and his assistants Margaret Knott and Dorothy Voss.

The "ring" portion of the name of this water therapy technique refers to the ring-shaped flotation devices used to support the client as they move across the water's surface. During the session, the client is lying supine in waist- or shoulder-deep water.

The Bad Ragaz Ring Method is commonly used with clients suffering from rheumatoid arthritis, soft tissue injuries, spinal injuries, head injuries and Parkinson's disease. Fibromyalgia sufferers may also find relief from their chronic pain by incorporating this form of treatment into their overall plan of care.

Burdenko Method of Hydrotherapy

The Burdenko Method was created by a Soviet professor of sports medicine, Igor Burdenko. He designed this form of therapy as an integrated land and water approach. Dr. Igor Burdenko currently serves as the founder and President of the Burdenko Water and Sports Therapy Institute in Boston. His organization offers therapists an opportunity to be certified in this specific aquatic therapy technique.

The Burdenko Method is often used for treating sports-related injuries. It works to improve a client's speed, strength, flexibility, coordination, balance and endurance. Clients begin performing rehabilitative exercises in the water and progress to performing the exercises on land as their condition improves.

Halliwick Concept for Aqua Therapy

Originally developed by fluid mechanics engineer James McMillan in the 1940s and 1950s, this aquatic therapy method focuses on helping clients develop balance and core stability. McMillan's work with students at the Halliwick School for Girls with Disabilities in London helped teach swimming skills and general independence to physically disabled young people.

The Halliwick Ten Point Programme includes:

- Mental adjustment.

- Sagittal rotation control.

- Transversal rotational control.

- Longitudinal rotation control.

- Combined rotation control.

- Upthrust or mental inversion.

- Balance in stillness.

- Turbulent gliding.

- Simple progression.

- Basic Halliwick movement.

Halliwick aquatic therapy is classified as a problem-solving approach. Therapists work to analyze the specific limitations and abilities of each client before developing interventions that will result in maximum functional increases.

Watsu Water Therapy

Watsu was developed in the early 1980s at Harbin Hot Springs, California by Harold Dull. In this form of aquatic therapy, the therapist supports the client through a series of flowing movements and stretches designed to induce deep relaxation as well as provide various therapeutic benefits. The movements combine elements of massage, shiatsu, dance, muscle stretching and joint mobilization.

Watsu is used to treat a wide range of orthopedic and neurological issues, either as a standalone therapy or a complement to a land-based therapeutic program. It has also served as the inspiration for other forms of aquatic therapy, including:

- Waterdance: This form of hydrotherapy was developed by Arjana Brunschwiler and Aman Schroter in 1987. It uses massage, rolls, inversions, dance, somersaults and Aikido-like moves. Clients begin the session with above water stretches and then progress to exercising underwater with a nose plug.

- Healing Dance: Combining elements of Watsu and Waterdance, Healing Dance was developed by Alexander Georgeakopoulos with a focus on flow, rhythm and 3D movements above and under the water.

- Jahara Technique: This peaceful form of aquatic therapy was developed by Mario Jahara and incorporates flotation devices to provide continued traction while stressing spinal alignment, muscular release and gentle bodywork.

Pool Therapy Exercises for Physical Fitness

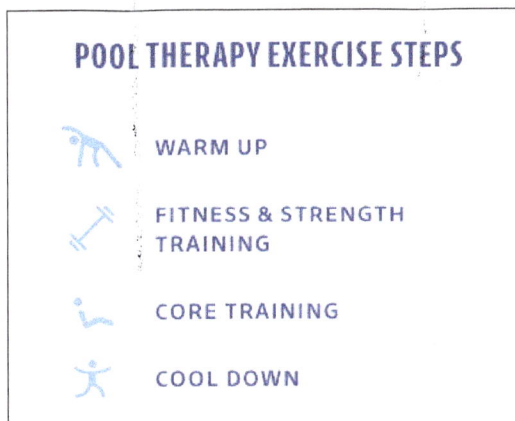

POOL THERAPY EXERCISE STEPS

WARM UP

FITNESS & STRENGTH TRAINING

CORE TRAINING

COOL DOWN

When aquatic therapy is intended to promote physical fitness, each session is broken into three parts:

- Warm up: The client begins with low-resistance exercises designed to target the upper and lower extremities. This often includes stretches and extensions, followed by brief walking or jogging on an underwater treadmill.

- Fitness and strength training: After the warm-up, the client will often perform cardiovascular activities such as running, sprint intervals or multi-planar activities. Strength activities, including plyometrics, can also be performed.

- Core training: After fitness and strength training, the client does 20-30 minutes of squats, leg swings, arm swings, shoulder presses and other core-training exercises.

- Cool down: Using a therapy pool with a massage hose attached to resistance jets provides a deep tissue massage experience that works muscles to prevent lactic acid buildup.

Types of Water Therapy Equipment

Treadmills for Underwater Running

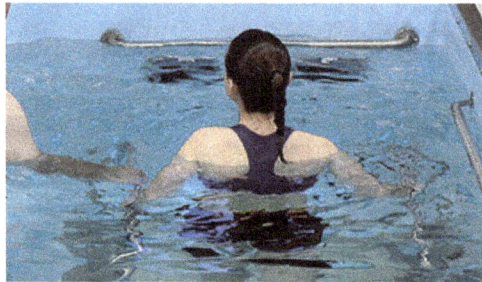

UNDERWATER TREADMILLS

The treadmills accelerate from **.1 mph to speeds of up to 10 mph**, making them suitable for everything from **walking and jogging to sprinting, side shuffling, backwards waking and carioca.**

Running provides an excellent cardiovascular workout, but can lead to joint damage. However, with an underwater treadmill, it's possible to enjoy all the benefits of running without the impact.

Underwater treadmills can be used to help athletes recover from injuries or to regain full-body motion after surgery. This is particularly useful if the athlete or patient is non or partial weight-bearing. High-end therapy pool models have resistance jets and adjustable speeds to allow for a gradual increase in workout intensity.

Benefits of using a treadmill as part of water therapy include:

- Promotes early range of motion.

- Initiates gait training in a low-impact environment.

- Duplicates land-based movement biomechanics to improve client's gait patterns more accurately than aqua jogging.

- Improves cardiovascular stamina.

- Impacts muscle strengthening.

- Increases ability to perform a wide range of plyometrics.

- Reduces blood pressure levels.

- Decreases joint stiffness.

- Offers the ability to perform exercises in multiple planes of motion.

Treadmills feature rubberized belts for extra traction and can be used with either bare feet or shoes. The treadmills accelerate from .1 mph to speeds of up to 10 mph, making them suitable for everything from walking and jogging to sprinting, side shuffling, backwards waking and carioca.

There are multiple types of aquatic therapy pools, ranging from small pools for single client use to large pools intended for group workouts. Therapists use cold-water plunge pools to speed muscle recovery in athletes and reduce joint inflammation. Hot-water plunge pools are used for relaxing muscles.

The newest models of therapy pools offer pinpoint temperature control and special massage hoses to target the specific muscles in need of treatment. A pool with underwater massage capabilities helps prevent lactic acid buildup, which reduces soreness and speeds recovery time. Massage can also provide an effective way to help people dealing with chronic pain.

Many therapy pools include stairs to promote safe accessibility for users with mobility issues. Therapists who frequently work with the elderly, small children or clients with serious injuries may utilize a pool with a moveable floor that makes it easier for clients to enter and exit the area.

Adjustable water depth controls, whether standard or as an optional therapy pool feature, benefit therapists by allowing for easy adjustments to pool water levels. This allows for a therapist to determine what percentage of the client's weight should be supported, creating a session that is tailored to the individual's abilities.

Underwater cameras are key features in effective aqua therapy pools, as they allow for therapists to monitor the client's form and progress from session to session or to make real-time adjustments. Clients can also use the cameras to provide an additional level of visual feedback as they work through a series of exercises.

Aqua Therapy Accessories

In addition to a functional therapy pool, accessories are sometimes used to enhance a specific exercise. Accessories might include:

- Stationary bicycles.

- Flotation rings or belts.

- Weight-adjustable barbells.

- Ankle weights.

- Short-tipped fins and flippers.

- Resistance bands and tubing.

- Resistance hand bells and paddles.

- Kickboards.

- Noodles.

The type of aqua therapy exercises a client needs will depend upon their required rehabilitation, physical limitations as well as the specific method of treatment. For example, the Bad Ragaz Ring Method relies on having the use of flotation rings around the client's neck, arms, pelvis and legs. For aqua jogging, a flotation belt is used to ensure the client remains in an upright position with their head above water.

Cognitive Rehabilitation Therapy

Cognitive Rehabilitation Therapy (CRT) is a broad term used to describe treatments that address the cognitive problems that can arise after a brain injury. Given the wide range of symptoms and severity of cognitive problems in individuals with brain injury, CRT does not refer to a specific approach to treatment. Although physical injuries, or speech or swallowing problems are typically covered by insurance, some health insurers deny coverage for CRT. Struggles with reimbursement may be due in part to the "invisible" nature of cognitive problems, but also to a lack of understanding about what CRT is.

Cognitive rehabilitation attempts to enhance functioning and independence in patients with cognitive impairments as a result of brain damage or disease, most commonly following TBI or stroke. It clarifies that CRT is different from cognitive behavioral therapy, a treatment approach for emotional and psychiatric problems. The IOM describes two broad approaches to CRT:

- Restorative treatment, whose goal is to improve the cognitive system to function in a wide range of activities.

- Compensatory treatment, which trains solutions to specific problem areas such as using memory notebooks or learning self-cuing strategies.

CRT has many variables: providers, settings, focus, and treatment formats. Many different types of professionals deliver services described as CRT. These providers are typically credentialed and licensed by their professions and state boards. They include, but may not be limited to:

- Speech-language pathologists.

- Occupational therapists.

- Physical therapists.

- Neuropsychologists.

- Vocational rehabilitation counsellors.

- Nurses.

- Physiatrists.

CRT services are provided in different settings, such as:

- Hospitals.

- Inpatient rehabilitation units.

- Outpatient departments.

- Community brain injury rehabilitation centers.

Treatment may also be delivered in a variety of formats (individual, group therapy, day treatment program), and intensities (intensive inpatient rehabilitation, daily outpatient, or weekly).

Accessing CRT

Ideally, cognitive assessment to evaluate level of alertness, orientation to surroundings, and memory of recent events begins from the moment someone with a brain injury is admitted to the hospital. With moderate or severe cognitive impairments, individuals may receive CRT during an inpatient rehabilitation program and then be discharged to an outpatient setting for further treatment. The treatment team and discharge coordinator typically make recommendations about the treatment setting and type of provider that will be most effective in working with the kinds of cognitive problems that the individual displays.

For example, someone with a moderate degree of cognitive impairment may benefit from a comprehensive outpatient CRT program that includes individual treatment as well as group therapy for social/behavioral goals. The program may include functional activities such as planning outings into the community, or work or school re-entry. Comprehensive programs like this may be staffed by providers from multiple disciplines.

More targeted therapy may be delivered by a single provider. For example, a person with cognitive issues related to language processing (following directions, using written strategies for memory and organization) may focus on speech-language pathology services. Someone working on the cognitive skills for driving or home management may receive occupational therapy. The professional who delivers the service may describe the treatment as CRT or in terms unique to that profession.

People who sustain a concussion or mild TBI without being hospitalized may have a more difficult time being referred for CRT and having treatment covered by insurance. Often the Emergency Room report doesn't describe cognitive problems, or the person doesn't notice difficulty concentrating or remembering until she returns to work or school. Without medical documentation of the problem, insurers may decline to make referrals or pay for CRT.

Challenging Insurance Denials for CRT

Because of the variability in patients and the CRT they may receive, research studies, to date, have not identified a single most effective treatment. In some cases, reports of limited research about CRT has led private health plans to deny CRT. The IOM report calls for more research on CRT, but recognizes the difficulty in obtaining conclusive results. The report states in italics "In fact, the committee supports the ongoing clinical application of CRT interventions for individuals with cognitive and behavioral deficits due to TBI."

Families and providers can work together to challenge insurance denials if they occur. Families can appeal denials, and ask the professional to provide detailed reports of functional progress made by the patient or articles demonstrating the effectiveness of the technique being used. Professional associations such as the American Speech-Language-Hearing Association provide assistance to speech-language pathologists and their patients by writing letters supporting CRT. Finally, appeals can be made to the state's Insurance Commission, where a review will take place at a level beyond the health plan.

Cognitive rehabilitation therapy may be like the proverbial elephant — it feels different to different people depending on their circumstances and perspective. But, as patients and families will attest, CRT is as fundamental a need in TBI recovery as physical rehabilitation and for some, even more essential to their quality of life.

Cardiac Rehabilitation

Cardiac rehabilitation refers to a structured program of exercise and education designed to help you return to optimal fitness and function following an event like a heart attack. It's usually provided by a team of specialists in various settings; these healthcare professionals work together to help you improve your functional mobility, decrease risk factors related to your cardiac injury, and help you and your family manage the psychosocial effects that may influence your recovery after a heart attack.

Physical therapists work as members of the cardiac rehabilitation team, helping to evaluate cardiac function, assess impairments that may limit your mobility, and prescribe progressive exercise and physical activity to help you return to your normal lifestyle after a cardiac event.

There are four phases of cardiac rehabilitation. The first phase occurs in the hospital after your cardiac event, and the other three phases occur in a cardiac rehab center or at home, once you've left the hospital. Keep in mind that the recovery after a cardiac event is variable; some people sail through each stage, while others may have a tough time getting back to normal. Work closely with your doctor to understand your progress and prognosis after a cardiac event.

Acute Phase

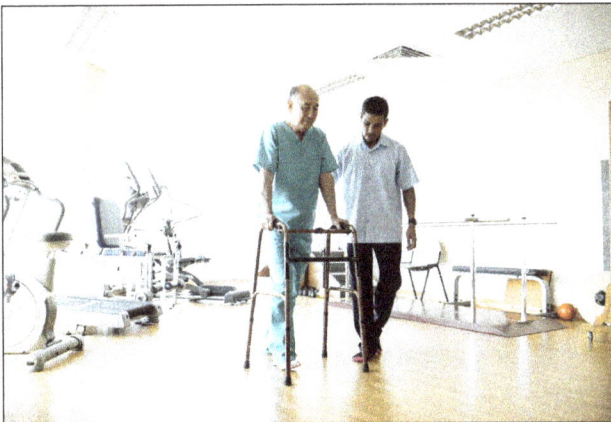

The initial phase of cardiac rehabilitation occurs soon after your cardiac event. An acute care physical therapist will work closely with your doctors, nurses, and other rehabilitation professionals to help you start to regain your mobility.

If you've had a severe cardiac injury or surgery, such as open-heart surgery, your physical therapist may start working with you in the intensive care unit (ICU). Once you no longer require the intensive monitoring and care of the ICU, you may be moved to a cardiac step down unit.

The initial goals of phase one cardiac rehabilitation include:

- Assess your mobility and the effects that basic functional mobility has on your cardiovascular system.

- Work with doctors, nurses and other therapists to ensure that appropriate discharge planning occurs.

- Prescribe safe exercises to help you improve your mobility, and to improve cardiac fitness.

- Help you maintain your sternal precautions is you have had open-heart surgery.

- Address any risk factors that may lead to cardiac events.

- Prescribe an appropriate assistive device, like a cane or a walker, to ensure that you are able to move around safely.

- Work with you and your family to provide education about your condition and the expected benefits and risks associated with a cardiac rehabilitation program.

Once significant healing has taken place, you may be discharged home to begin phase two cardiac rehab.

Subacute Phase

Once you leave the hospital, your cardiac rehabilitation program will continue at an outpatient facility. Phase two of cardiac rehabilitation usually lasts from three to six weeks and involves continued monitoring of your cardiac responses to exercise and activity.

Another important aspect of phase two cardiac rehabilitation is education about proper exercise procedures, and about how to self-monitor heart rate and exertion levels during exercise. This phase centers around your safe return to functional mobility while monitoring your heart rate.

Towards the end of phase two, you should be ready to begin more independent exercise and activity.

Intensive Outpatient Therapy

Phase three of cardiac rehabilitation involves more independent and group exercise. You should be able to monitor your own heart rate, your symptomatic response to exercise, and your rating of perceived exertion (RPE). Your physical therapist will be present during this phase to help you increase your exercise tolerance and to monitor any negative changes that may occur during this phase of cardiac rehab.

As you become more and more independent during phase three of cardiac rehabilitation, your physical therapist can help tailor a program of exercises, including flexibility, strengthening, and aerobic exercise.

Independent Ongoing Conditioning

The final phase of cardiac rehabilitation is your own independent and ongoing conditioning. If you have participated fully in the previous three phases, then you should have excellent knowledge about your specific condition, risk factors, and strategies to maintain optimal health.

Independent exercise and conditioning are essential to maintaining optimal health and preventing possible future cardiac problems. While phase four is an independent maintenance phase, your physical therapist is available to help make changes to your current exercise routine to help you achieve physical fitness and wellness.

An unexpected cardiac event, like a heart attack or open-heart surgery, can be a scary and life-altering experience. By working closely with your doctor and rehab team, and by participating fully in the four phases of cardiac rehabilitation, you can increase your chances of returning to optimal health quickly and safely.

Robotic Neurorehabilitation

Neurological disorders leave most with devastating disabilities such as the loss of movement in an arm or leg, and the accompanying loss of freedom of movement. Initially, these disabilities were considered incurable and therapy often focused on training people to use their "good side."

Fortunately research shows that the concept of "task-specific learning", in Neurorehabilitation based on neuroplasticity, suggests that activities of daily living may be trained and improved through continuous repetition in neurological patients. Robotic therapy meets this demand and enables intensive functional locomotion therapy with augmented feedback.

Robotics has come a long way in the past few years, and while we're not yet creating bionic men and women, we can at least claim to make people "better, stronger, and faster."

Robotics can compensate for the patient's inadequate strength or motor control at speeds individually calibrated on the residual motor functions, while continuous feedback provides the patient with subjective perception of improvement. These characteristics make robotics a potential support in the rehabilitation domain for both trainers and patients, whose role remains central to the process. Robotic Neurorehabilitation is attractive because of its potential for easy deployment, its applicability across of a wide range of motor impairment, and its high measurement reliability.

Lokomat

While two-thirds of people who suffer from a neurological condition regain ambulatory function, the resulting gait pattern is typically asymmetrical, slow, and metabolically inefficient, mostly associated with difficulty in advancing and bearing weight through the more affected limb, leading to instability, along with increased risk of falls. Secondary impairments, including muscle disuse and reduced cardiorespiratory capacity, often contribute to further functional declines in gait. Hence, improved walking is one of the most frequently articulated goals of rehabilitation and interventions that effectively enhance locomotor function. They are essential in the rehabilitation of neurological patients following stroke, spinal cord injury, and traumatic brain injury, as well as in patients with multiple sclerosis, cerebral palsy or other neurological disorders.

Lokomat consists of a driven robotic gait orthosis that guides the patient's legs on a treadmill offering a wide range of training possibilities and has a pre-programmed gait pattern facilitating a bilaterally symmetrical gait pattern as the individual actively attempts to advance each limb while walking on the treadmill. The pre-programmed walking pattern corresponds with normal gait kinematics including: gait cycle timing (i.e. stance vs. swing phase), inter-limb and inter-joint coordination, appropriate limb loading, and afferent signalling. Lokomat can be used in both adult and paediatric population likewise.

Lokomat entails the following benefits:

- Faster progress through longer and more intensive functional training sessions compared to manual treadmill training with adjustable level of difficulty and intensity according to the cognitive abilities and the specific needs of each patient.

- Patient walking activity is easily supervised and assessed.

- Gait pattern and guidance force are individually adjustable to the patient's needs to optimize the functional training.

- Improved patient motivation through visualized performance feedback offering various engaging virtual environments.

- Assessment tools allow easy and reproducible measurements of the patient's progress

- If needed - easily switch from automated to manual therapy.

- An integrated biofeedback system monitors the patient's gait and provides real-time visual performance feedback to motivate the patient for active participation.

Erigo

Accelerates early rehabilitation and minimizes complications of debilitated/bedridden and neurologically impaired patients.

Patients confined to prolonged bed rest endure reduced cardiac output, reduced oxygen uptake, muscle atrophy and skeletal demineralization, and the risk of injury when eventually elevated.

The Erigo combines a continuously adjustable tilt table with a robotic stepping mechanism, enabling early, intensive therapy.

- Combines three established therapies in one-verticalization, leg movement, and cyclic loading and unloading of lower extremities.

- Supports and facilitates patient mobilization.

- Provides intensive afferent sensory stimulation.

- Activates the cardiovascular system.

- Repetitive physical motion reduces spasticity in some patients.

- May reduce risk of secondary complications caused by immobility.

- May improve alertness in vegetative state patients.

Armeo

The Armeo Therapy Concept improves the efficiency of therapy treatments because the exercises are self-initiated, self-directed, functional and intense. Even severely impaired patients can practice independently, without the constant presence of a therapist, allowing patients to explore their full potential for recovery.

The Armeo's purpose is to support functional therapy for patients who have lost the function of or have restricted function in their upper extremities caused by cerebral, neurogenic, spinal, muscular or bone-related disorders.

The Augmented Feedback provided by the shared software platform:

- Encourages and motivates patients to achieve a higher number of repetitions, and this leads to better, faster results and improved long-term outcomes.

- Provides adjustable difficulty levels according to the patient's needs and progress.

- Provides adjustable workspace according to the patients' changing abilities The "Continuum of Rehabilitation", from immediate post-injury to long-term recovery, requires a range of therapies to address the changing needs of the recovering patient.

References

- Chest-Physical-Therapy, Treatments-and-Therapies-Airway-Clearance: cff.org, Retrieved 03 February, 2019

- Orthopedic-physical-therapy-4013256: verywellhealth.com, Retrieved 16 June, 2019

- Geriatric-therapy, medical-rehabilitation-therapy: disabled-world.com, Retrieved 08 January, 2019

- Neurological-physical-therapy: aptclinics.com, Retrieved 02 February, 2019

- Aquatic-therapy-guide, research-education-additional-resources: hydroworx.com, Retrieved 19 June, 2019

- What-about-cognitive-rehabilitation-therapy: brainline.org, Retrieved 05 March, 2019

- Four-phases-of-cardiac-rehabilitation-2696089: verywellhealth.com, Retrieved 18 August, 2019

Chapter 3

Neuromuscular Medicine

Neuromuscular medicine is the product of amalgamation of neurology and physiatry which plays a vital role in the treatment of neuromuscular diseases. Some of the important areas covered in this field are neuromuscular diseases and rehabilitation, myotonic dystrophy, etc. The topics elaborated in this chapter will help in gaining a better perspective about neuromuscular medicine.

Neuromuscular Disorders

The brain controls the movements of skeletal (voluntary) muscles via specialised nerves. The combination of the nervous system and muscles, working together to permit movement, is known as the neuromuscular system.

If you want to move part of your body, a message is sent to particular neurons (nerve cells), called upper motor neurons. Upper motor neurons have long tails (axons) that go into and through the brain, and into the spinal cord, where they connect with lower motor neurons. At the spinal cord, the lower motor neurons in the spinal cord send their axons via nerves in the arms and legs directly to the muscle they control.

A typical muscle is serviced by anywhere between 50 and 200 (or more) lower motor neurons. Each lower motor neuron is subdivided into many tiny branches. The tip of each branch is called a presynaptic terminal. This connection between the tip of the nerve and the muscle is also called the neuromuscular junction.

The electrical signal from the brain travels down the nerves and prompts the release of the chemical acetylcholine from the presynaptic terminals. This chemical is picked up by special sensors (receptors) in the muscle tissue. If enough receptors are stimulated by acetylcholine, your muscles will contract.

There are many diseases that are classified as neuromuscular disorders.

Symptoms of Neuromuscular Disorders

The symptoms of neuromuscular disease vary according to the condition and may be mild, moderate or life threatening. The following are symptoms.

- Muscular Weakness,

- Muscle wastage,

- Muscular cramps,

- Muscle spasticity (stiffness), which later causes joint or skeletal deformities,

- Muscle pain,

- Breathing difficulties,

- Swallowing difficulties.

Causes of Neuromuscular Disorders

Some of the causes may include:

- Genetic mutation,

- Viral infection,

- Autoimmune disorder,

- Hormonal disorder,

- Metabolic disorder,

- Dietary deficiency,

- Certain drugs and poisons,

- Unknown factors.

Classifications of Neuromuscular Disorders

Some of the major diseases which affect the neuromuscular system are classified into four main groups, including:

- Motor neurone diseases: For unknown or genetic reasons, the lower (and sometimes also the upper) motor neurons gradually die. Some of the different types of genetic (inherited) motor neuron diseases include infantile progressive spinal muscular atrophy (SMA1), intermediate spinal muscular atrophy (SMA2), juvenile spinal muscular atrophy (SMA3) and adult spinal muscular atrophy. The most common form of motor neuron disease, known simply as motor neurone disease or amyotrophic lateral sclerosis or Lou Gehrig's disease, is usually not inherited and its cause remains unknown.

- Neuropathies: The peripheral nervous system (nerves other than those within the spinal cord) is affected. Some of the different diseases of the peripheral nerve include the genetic disease Charcot-Marie-Tooth disease, the hormonal disorder diabetes (if poorly controlled), and autoimmune diseases such as chronic inflammatory demyelinating neuropathy (CIDP).

- Neuromuscular junction disorders: In these diseases, the transmission of the signal to move (contract) a muscle is blocked as it tries to bridge the gap between the nerve and muscle. The most common of these diseases is myasthenia gravis, an autoimmune disease where the immune system produces antibodies that attach themselves to the neuromuscular junction and prevent transmission of the nerve impulse to the muscle.

- Myopathies including muscular dystrophies: Many different types of muscular dystrophy (muscle wastage) are caused by various genetic mutations that prevent the maintenance and repair of muscle tissue. Some of the different types include Becker muscular dystrophy, congenital muscular dystrophy, Duchenne muscular dystrophy and facioscapulohumeral muscular dystrophy. Other diseases of the muscles (myopathies) can be caused as a rare side effect of medications (for example, the cholesterol-lowering drugs known as statins), autoimmune disease such as polymyositis or polymyalgia rheumatica or hormonal disorders such as hypothyroidism.

Types of Neuromuscular Disorders

A neuromuscular disorder is a term that encompasses many different medical conditions that impair the functioning of the muscles.

Arthrogryposis

Arthrogryposis (also called arthrogryposis multiplex congenital or AMC) is a congenital non-progressive neuromuscular disorder characterized by stiffness and limited range of motion in two or more joints. Joint contractures which cause the limited range of motion develop before birth (prenatally) and are evident at birth (congenitally).

Any and all joints can be affected, but it is possible for some joints to be unaffected. No two people are affected the same way. Treatment often includes stretching, range of motion exercises, splinting, serial casting, physical therapy, occupational therapy and bracing.

Arthrogryposis has been estimated to occur once in every 3,000 live births. It is not thought to be a genetic or hereditary condition. Currently, the exact cause is unknown.

Autosomal Recessive Spastic Ataxia of Charlevoix-Saguenay (Arsacs)

Autosomal recessive spastic ataxia of Charlevoix-Saguenay (ARSACS) is a hereditary progressive neurological disorder that mainly affects people from the Saguenay-Lac-St-Jean (SLS) and Charlevoix regions as well as people whose ancestors are from these areas. There are approximately 250 people from the Charlevoix-Saguenay region who are living with this progressive disorder.

The condition, which can affect both males and females, is characterized by degeneration of the spinal cord and progressive damage of the peripheral nerves. Children are usually diagnosed at a young age with symptoms such as poor motor coordination, spastic stiffness, muscle wasting, and slurred speech. These symptoms worsen over time, leaving most patients unable to walk by their early 40s and with a reduced life expectancy.

ARSACS is caused by a gene mutation located on chromosome 13. It is estimated that one out of every 22 people from SLSJ are carriers of the mutated gene.

Becker Muscular Dystrophy

Becker muscular dystrophy (BMD) is an inherited degenerative muscle disorder that occurs almost exclusively in males. BMD is similar to DMD — both are caused by a mutation in the dystrophin gene on the X chromosome. This protein is an important building block that helps give muscles structure and strength.

Both DMD and BMD primarily affect skeletal muscles, which are used for movement, and heart (cardiac) muscle. However, BMD is less common — 1 in 35,000 males worldwide — and has a later onset and slower progression than DMD.

Symptoms typically appear between the ages of five and 15 and include difficulty with: walking; rising from the floor; running; hopping and/or jumping.

Charcot-Marie-Tooth Disease

Charcot-Marie-Tooth (CMT) disease is an inherited peripheral neuropathy. Inherited means that something can be passed on from generation to generation. Neuropathy means that there is a problem with the nerves. Peripheral refers to the peripheral nervous system, which is all of the nerves that branch from the central nervous system (brain and spinal cord) and travel to the feet and hands — the periphery of the body.

People with CMT usually have problems with their feet and hands, including feet deformity (high arches and hammertoes), foot drop, abnormal sensations and loss of fine motor skills. Not everyone with CMT is affected in the same way. Some patients have mild neuropathy, while others may have more severe problems with walking, hands, and/or sensation.

CMT occurs in both men and women and can affect children and adults. There is no known predisposition to having CMT based on race or ethnicity. CMT is a genetic condition. For a person to be affected with CMT, that person must have one (or two, depending on the type of CMT) disease causing mutation in one of the genes that causes CMT. There are at least forty different genes that cause CMT when mutated. A mutation in any one of them can cause the disease.

The diagnosis of CMT is made by combining clinical features with a nerve conduction study, which is a test where an electrical signal is sent down the nerve. CMT is an inherited peripheral neuropathy — a person must have a peripheral neuropathy based on a nerve conduction test in order to be affected with the condition. Genetic testing can also be done in order to identify a specific sub-type of CMT. Once a sub-type is identified in the family, other family members may just need the nerve conduction or the genetic testing in order to determine if that person is also affected.

Treatment of CMT is supportive. Ambulation aids, such as foot orthotics and braces (anke-foot-orthotics, AFOs) are commonly needed to help with foot deformity and foot drop. Surgery to correct foot alignment or to lengthen or transfer tendons is often performed. Physical and occupational therapies are instrumental in providing long-lasting quality of life. There is no cure for CMT nor any drug or vitamin known at this time to improve CMT symptoms.

Congenital Muscular Dystrophy

Congenital muscular dystrophy (CMD) is the name for a group of muscular dystrophies that are united by the fact that muscle weakness begins in infancy or in early childhood (typically before age 2). Sometimes, the condition is not detected until a child is found to have trouble with certain developmental milestones — such as learning to walk. Both boys and girls can develop CMD. There are several different types of CMD, which have different symptoms, degrees of severity, and rates of progression.

Duchenne Muscular Dystrophy

Duchenne Muscular dystrophy (DMD) is an inherited disorder, which usually affects boys (it is very rare in girls). The muscles become weaker as boys get older. This is because the body cannot make the muscle protein called dystrophin. This makes the muscle cells weak and they gradually break down. Signs of weakness start when the boys are between 3 and 5 years of age (sometimes earlier). At first, the weakness is seen mostly in the legs and hips. The children may:

- Fall frequently.

- Have trouble running as fast as their peers.

- Have trouble climbing stairs.

- Have trouble getting up from a chair.

- Develop big calves.

- Frequently walk on their toes and lean backwards to keep their balance.

Eventually this weakness also makes walking more difficult and a wheelchair is needed. Gradually, all the muscles become very weak, including the muscles used for breathing and the heart.

Anaesthesia or Sedation Risks

The American College of Chest Physicians issued a consensus statement on the management of patients with DMD undergoing anaesthesia or sedation.

Thanks to better cardiac and respiratory care, patients with Duchenne muscular dystrophy (DMD) are living longer than in the past. Increased lifespan means it is more likely that DMD patients will undergo surgical procedures. Therefore, it is important to be aware of the risks and guidelines for patient care during and after surgery.

- Consider using intravenous, rather than gas, anaesthetics.

- Do not use depolarizing muscle relaxants, such as succinylcholine; fatal reactions can occur.

- Have an intensive care unit available for postoperative care.

- Provide respiratory support during anaesthesia or sedation, using any of a variety of techniques.

- Monitor blood oxygen saturation using pulse oximeter throughout the procedure.

- When possible, monitor blood or lung carbon dioxide levels.

- Consider moving the patient from intubation (tube in the trachea) during surgery to non-invasive positive pressure ventilation right after surgery.

- Use extreme caution when administering supplemental oxygen.

- Use manually assisted cough and insufflation-exsufflation assisted cough postoperatively to clear secretions.

- Obtain a cardiology consultation, and closely monitor cardiac and fluid status postoperatively.

- Initiate bowel regimens to avoid and treat constipation.

- Consider gastric (stomach) decompression with a nasogastric tube.

- Start intravenous feeding or enteral (through the stomach and intestines) tube feeding if oral intake is delayed for more than 24 to 48 hours postoperatively.

Respiratory Care

The statement recommends that physicians caring for patients with DMD should provide:

- Baseline respiratory status evaluation early in the disease course (between ages 4 and 6).

- Regular consultations with a physician specializing in pediatric respiratory care twice a year after starting wheelchair use, reaching a vital capacity (maximal amount of air that can be exhaled after a maximal inhalation) that's below 80 percent of predicted (normal), or reaching age 12.

- Consultations every three to six months after starting mechanically assisted ventilation or airway clearance device.

- Tests to evaluate pulmonary function at each clinic visit.

- Education about assisted ventilation options well before an emergency occurs.

- Nutritional guidance and support, including the placement of a feeding (gastrostomy) tube when indicated.

- Regular evaluations of sleep quality and sleep-disordered breathing.

- Regular cardiac evaluations, including annual electrocardiograms and echocardiograms, starting at least by school age.

- Regular evaluations of the ability to clear secretions (cough).

- Manually assisted cough techniques or mechanical cough assistance with an insufflator-exsufflator (positive and negative pressure) device when secretion clearance becomes less than adequate.

- Education in the use of pulse oximetry (measurement of the amount of oxygen in the blood through the skin, via a painless sensor) at home to monitor the effectiveness of airway clearance.

- Non-invasive ventilatory support via nasal intermittent positive pressure ventilation, either with a bi-level (using different pressures for inhalation and exhalation) airway pressure device, or with a mechanical ventilator, when disrupted or inadequate breathing during sleep or low blood oxygen levels during sleep are detected.

- Avoidance of supplemental oxygen to treat sleep-related hypoventilation (inadequate breathing) unless ventilatory assistance is also being used.

- Non-invasive daytime ventilation when breathing becomes inadequate during the day, using intermittent positive pressure ventilation through a mouthpiece, or an inflatable bladder that provides intermittent abdominal pressure simulating breathing.

- Education in glossopharyngeal breathing (a "gulping" type of breathing) to use during short periods when off mechanical ventilation.

- The option of ventilation via tracheostomy (surgical opening into the trachea in the neck) if non-invasive ventilation isn't feasible or isn't desired, with appropriate education for the patient and family.

- Avoidance of preventive (before required) mechanically assisted ventilation, unless and until it is proven useful, since it may lead to a false sense of security and inadequate respiratory function monitoring.

- Evaluation of pulmonary and cardiac function and of breathing during sleep before scoliosis surgery, and airway clearance and respiratory support in the postoperative period.

- The option of oral steroid therapy with prednisone or deflazacort as a possible means to preserve lung function.

- Education about respiratory function and treatment, including end-of-life care options, for the patient and family.

- End-of-life care that includes treatment of pain or difficulty breathing, while attending to the psychosocial and spiritual needs of the patient and family and respecting their choices concerning tests and treatments.

Facioscapularhumeral Muscular Dystrophy

Facioscapulohumeral muscular dystrophy (FSH or FSHD) is an inherited muscle disorder that causes progressive breakdown of muscle fibres, resulting in muscle atrophy and weakness. FSHD is the third most common muscular dystrophy worldwide, after Duchenne muscular dystrophy and myotonic dystrophy, affecting approximately 1 in 20,000 individuals.

Symptoms typically begin in teenage years, predominantly affecting the face (facio), shoulder blades (scapular), upper arm (humeral), and legs. There are currently no treatments to slow down, stop, or reverse the symptoms of FSHD.

Friedrich's Ataxia

Friedreich's ataxia (FA) is a genetic neuromuscular disorder characterized by spinocerebellar degeneration. People with FA have gene mutations that limit the production of frataxin, which is an important protein that functions in the mitochondria (energy producing factories) of the cell. Additionally, in FA, specific nerve cells (neurons) degenerate, which is directly manifested in FA symptoms.

FA affects approximately 1 in 40,000 people. Childhood onset of FA is usually between the ages of 5 and 15, and is often associated with rapid progression. Late onset FA can occur anytime during adulthood.

FA symptoms may include:

- Loss of arm and leg coordination,

- Fatigue,

- Muscle loss,

- Vision impairment,

- Hearing loss,

- Slurred speech,

- Aggressive scoliosis (curvature of the spine),

- Diabetes mellitus,

- And a serious heart condition.

The mental capabilities of people with FA are unaffected.

Guillain Barré Syndrome

Guillain-Barré syndrome (GBS) is an inflammatory disorder of the (located outside the brain and spinal cord) which are attacked by the body's immune system. These damaged nerves are unable, to varying degrees, to perform their functions correctly. The reason for the immune system's attack on the body is currently unknown. However, the focus of the attack is the myelin sheath that surrounds the axons of nerve cells and sometimes, the axons themselves.

GBS is considered a rare disorder, affecting approximately 2 to 3 per 100,000 people a year. The incidence tends to increase with age, so GBS is most common in people between the ages of 50 and 80.

Most often, GBS follows a viral or bacterial infection, but pregnancy, surgery, or vaccinations may trigger the disorder in rare instances. GBS symptoms may include: lower limb numbness and tingling, symmetrical leg and arm weakness, severe back pain, muscle aching and cramping, shortness of breath and bieralfacial drooping (palsy). Severity of symptoms can vary greatly from person to person.

Symmetrical leg and arm weakness helps differentiate GBS from other disorders.

GBS treatment may include plasmapheresis (plasma exchange), immunoglobulin therapy, assisted ventilation and occupational therapy.

Hereditary Motor and Sensory Neuropathy with Agenesis of the Corpus Callosum

Hereditary Motor and Sensory Neuropathy with Agenesis of the Corpus Callosum (HMSN/ACC) is a progressive hereditary neuromuscular disorder that mainly affects people from the Saguenay-Lac-St-Jean (SLSJ) and Charlevoix regions of Quebec as well as people whose ancestors originated from these regions. Some cases of HMSN/ACC have also been identified in other countries.

HMSN/ACC is responsible for the degeneration of the peripheral nerves involved in both body movement and the perception of sensations. Irregularities are observed in the brain of people affected with HMSN/ACC, mainly in the anatomical structure connecting the two cerebral hemispheres known as the corpus callosum. The corpus callosum is completely absent in 57.8% of patients and partially absent in 9.4% of patients. The presence or absence of corpus callosum in the brain of people affected does not seem to influence the severity or nature of symptoms. Men and women are equally affected.

HMSN/ACC is an autosomal recessive genetic disorder. It is caused by a gene mutation located on chromosome 15, one of the 22 autosomal pairs of chromosomes. The gene is expressed (resulting in the manifestation of HMSN/ACC) only when it is inherited from both parents. This means that both parents must be carriers of the gene. Often, carriers of the HMSN/ACC gene do not have symptoms and do not know that they are carriers.

When both parents are carriers of the HMSN/ACC gene, at each pregnancy:

- There is a 1 in 4 (25%) chance that the child will have the disorder.

- There is a 2 in 4 (50%) chance that the child will be a carrier of the gene.

- There is a 1 in 4 (25%) chance that the child will neither have the disorder nor be a carrier of the gene.

The carrier status of the HMSN/ACC gene can be confirmed through genetic testing. If you have a family history of HMSN/ACC, you may wish to consult a genetic counselor to understand your chances of having a child affected with HMSN/ACC and discuss family planning alternatives.

A paediatrician and/or neurologist will conduct a clinical examination, as well as genetic testing to confirm diagnosis of HMSN/ACC. Additional testing may be recommended, such as a brain scan performed with highly precise radiography technology (cerebral tomography) or an analysis of the electrical activity in the arm and leg muscles (electromyogram).

Symptoms appear shortly after birth or during the first year of life and are characterized by a lack of muscle strength and a delay in the development of motor skills. HMSN/ACC results in a loss of mobility and developmental abnormalities in the spine, hands, and feet. In addition to the physical symptoms, HMSN/ACC also causes mild to moderate cognitive impairment.

Babies with HMSN/ACC have difficulty sitting and crawling. An intensive physiotherapy and occupational therapy treatment can stimulate motor development. With the use of assistive devices, such as feet and ankle orthoses, walkers, quadripods or support canes, toddlers usually begin to walk around the age of two or three. Typically, a child affected with HMSN/ACC has a slow gait and poor balance. In most cases, tremors are experienced throughout all parts of the body.

Children with HMSN/ACC experience delays in gross and fine motor development. Young children will be less prone to use their arms. Handgrip strength is weak, and keeping a grip on an object often requires extra exertion. Sometimes, this weakness in the upper limbs will cause muscle tremors when under strain. Often, children with HMSN/ACC are hypersensitive to touch. They are rarely toilet trained before the age of three.

Language development is delayed and learning capacity is affected. Students with HMSN/ACC usually require the support of a teaching assistant, or may be placed in a specialized class. Most children with HMSN/ACC learn to read, write, and count and are able to acquire general knowledge. However, skills typically remain at a second grade level.

Children with HMSN/ACC are usually very sociable, affectionate, and cheerful, and are able to integrate well in school and group activities. Additionally, they are able to follow codes of conduct and demonstrate social and moral judgment.

Around the age of twelve, the orthopedic surgeon may recommend scoliosis surgery to correct the curvature or bending of the spine. This surgery allows for a better expansion of the lungs and other organs as well as a better body alignment. Prior to the surgery, some children wear a corset for a few years to minimize the curvature of the spine or delay of the surgery. However, the corset is not a substitute for the surgery.

With the help of a walker, some people with HMSN/ACC will be able to walk until their early twenties. Many teenagers, however, will use a manual wheelchair or an electric scooter for mobility.

By the end of the teenage years or at the beginning of adulthood, some people may experience episodes of anxiety, agitation, visual or auditory hallucinations or depression. These problems are caused by dysfunctions in the brain and may require treatment.

Due to the progressive nature of the disorder, the person affected typically requires a power wheelchair and assistance with their personal needs by early twenties. Respiratory muscle weakness results in a high risk of respiratory failure and bronchopneumonia, which can be fatal. The average life span is 29 years, although many have lived up to their forties.

Currently, there is no known cure for HMSN/ACC or treatments to prevent the onset of symptoms. However, therapeutic interventions offered by various health care providers may help maintain physical abilities, avoid further complications and enhance comfort.

Limb Girdle Muscular Dystrophy

Limb-girdle muscular dystrophy (LGMD) is an inherited group of disorders that cause arm and leg muscle weakness and atrophy. The muscles most affected are those closest to the body (proximal muscles), specifically the shoulder, upper arm, pelvic and thigh muscles. Occasionally, the heart (cardiac) and breathing (respiratory) muscles may be affected. There are many subtypes of LGMD, including some that don't have LGMD in their name, such as Bethlem myopathy, desmin myopathy, dysferlinopathy, myofibrillar myopathy, sarcoglycanopathies and ZASP-related myopathy. As of late 2012, there are more than 20 different LGMD subtypes, which is a complex and continuously evolving area of research.

LGMD incidence ranges from 1 in 14,500 to 1 in 123,000 individuals. The various LGMD forms are caused by mutations in many different genes. These genes provide instructions for making proteins that are involved in muscle maintenance and repair.

The severity, age of onset, and features of LGMD vary among the many subtypes. Early symptoms may include: difficulty walking, running, and rising from the floor. LGMD treatment may include: physical and occupational therapy, assistive devices, physiotherapy, orthoses and surgery.

Mcardle's Disease

Also known as Glycogen Storage Disease Type V (GSD V), Phosphorylase Deficiency, and Myophosphorylase Deficiency.

McArdle's disease is an inherited condition that affects the skeletal muscles, causing severe muscle pain and cramping. It is caused by the lack of an enzyme called phosphorylase or myophosphorylase, which is needed to break down glycogen (stored form of sugar). Without the enzyme, glycogen can't be used to produce energy during exercise.

McArdle's disease is rare, and its prevalence is unknown. The condition is present from birth, but may not be diagnosed until young adulthood. People with McArdle's disease often report they had symptoms, such as painful muscle spasms, during childhood. Treatment may include physiotherapy and regular moderate exercise (i.e. walking).

Some anaesthetics used during surgery can cause acute muscle damage or other complications. You should notify the surgeon and/or the anesthesiologist that you have been diagnosed with McArdle's disease prior to receiving any anaesthetics.

Mitochondrial Myopathy

Mitochondrial myopathy affects the mitochondria — the tiny energy-producing structures that serve as "power plants of the cell."

The term refers to a group of muscle disorders, including:

- Kearns-Sayre syndrome (KSS)

  ◦ Leigh's syndrome,

  ◦ Mitochondrial Depletion syndrome (MDS),

  ◦ Mitochondrial Encephalomyopathy,

  ◦ Lactic Acidosis and Stroke-like episodes (MELAS),

  ◦ Myoclonic epilepsy with Ragged Red Fibers (MERRG),

  ◦ Mitochondrial neurogastrointestinal encephalopathy syndrome (MNGIE),

  ◦ Neuropathy, Ataxia, and Retinitis Pigmentosa (NARP),

  ◦ Pearson syndrome,

  ◦ Chronic Progressive External Opthalmoplegia (CPEO).

Some types of mitochondrial myopathy are inherited, while some are sporadic (the mutation only occurs in the affected person; it was not inherited and will not be passed onto children). These disorders are caused by a defect in either a mitochondrial gene or a gene in the cell nucleus that affects the functioning of the mitochondria.

Symptoms may include:

- Nervous system impairment,

- Eye problems,

- Hearing issues,

- Cardiac irregularities,

- Skeletal muscle abnormalities,

- Gastrointestinal tract disorders,

- Muscle weakness and pain,

- Fatigue,

- Lack of endurance,

- Poor balance,

- Difficulty swallowing.

Treatment may include:

- Hearing aids,

- Medication,

- Surgery,

- Specialized glasses,

- Assistive devices,

- Speech therapy,

- Diet modification,

- Respiratory support.

Some patients report minor improvement in symptoms when taking a supplement "cocktail" of Creatine, L-carnitine, and coenzyme Q10.

Multicore Myopathy

Multicore myopathy (MM) or Multi Minicore myopathy causes muscle fibre degeneration. Most cases of MM are inherited, but some are sporadic (the mutation only occurs in the affected person; it was not inherited and will not be passed onto children).

There are four types of MM:

- Classic form,

- Progressive form with hand involvement,

- Antenatal form with arthrogryposis multiplex congenital,

- Ophthalmoplegic form.

MM affects both males and females. Close to half of MM cases are caused by a defective gene in one of two proteins: Selenprotein N1 (SEPN1) and Ryanodine receptor 1 (RYR1).

The main symptoms of MM are generalized weakness and muscle atrophy. Other symptoms depend on the type of MM. In some people, the disorder may remain stable for a long period of time, while some may experience progressive muscle weakness.

Myasthenia Gravis

Myasthenia gravis (MG) is an autoimmune disorder that produces weakness and irregularly rapid fatigue of voluntary muscles. In MG, the immune system attacks the body; the acetylcholine (ACH) receptor sites at the neuromuscular junction (point where the nerve endings join the muscle surface) are the targets.

MG affects approximately 20 per 100,000 people worldwide. Currently, the cause of MG is unknown. The disorder is seldom fatal, though it can be life-threatening in situations where muscle weakness interferes with respiration (breathing).

The first noticeable symptom is often eye muscle weakness, resulting in droopy eyelids (ptosis) or double vision (diplopia).

Other symptoms may include:

- Weakness in muscles used for chewing, swallowing and talking,

- Severe fatigue,

- An unstable or waddling gait,

- Arm weakness resulting in an inability to raise the arms over the head,

- Hand and finger weakness,

- Breathing difficulty.

Myositis Disorders

Myositis disorders are autoimmune conditions characterized by voluntary (skeletal) muscle inflammation. The primary symptom of these disorders is muscle weakness, which is usually progressive and may be severely impairing.

There are three main types:

- Polymyositis: Inflammation is found in many muscles,

- Inclusion body myositis: Muscle is characterized by irregular inclusions—accumulations of misfolded protein,

- Dermatomyositis: Muscle inflammation is accompanied by a skin rash.

All three conditions are considered rare. The cause of each of these disorders is currently unknown. Each of these disorders greatly differs in response to treatment.

Myotonia Congenita

Myotonia congenita is an inherited condition that affects muscle relaxation. It is congenital, meaning that it is present from birth.

The two major types of myotonia congenita are known as Thomsen disease and Becker disease. These conditions are distinguished by the severity of their symptoms and their patterns of inheritance.

Abnormal repeated electrical signals occur in the muscles, causing a stiffness called myotonia.

Although myotonia can affect any skeletal muscles, including muscles of the face and tongue, it occurs most often in the legs. Myotonia causes muscle stiffness that can interfere with movement. In some people the stiffness is very mild, while in other cases it may be severe enough to interfere with walking, running, and other activities of daily life. These muscle problems are particularly noticeable during movement following a period of rest. Many affected individuals find that repeated movements can temporarily alleviate their muscle stiffness, a phenomenon known as the warm-up effect.

Myotonia congenita has been estimated to occur once in every 100,000 people worldwide.

Myotonic Dystrophy

Myotonic dystrophy is the most common form of adult-onset muscular dystrophy, with a worldwide prevalence of 14 per 100,000 population and 189 per 100,000 population in Saguenay-Lac-Saint-Jean region of Quebec. Myotonic dystrophy is an autosomal dominant disorder caused by an error in genes located on chromosome 19 or chromosome 3.

There are two types of myotonic dystrophy:

- Type 1, also known as Steinert's disease,

- Type 2, also known as proximal myotonic myopathy (PROMM) – is caused by a mutation in the CNBP gene. This type is only found in adults, with an age of onset generally between 30 and 60 years.

Symptoms include:

- Myotonia that results in a delay in the ability to relax the muscles after a prolonged contraction,

- Voluntary muscle weakness,

- Muscle stiffness,

- Drooping eyelids,

- Unclear word pronunciation,

- Difficulty raising the head when lying down,

- Difficulty holding an object firmly,

- A shuffling gait,

- Difficulty climbing stairs or rising from a seated position.

Nemaline Myopathy

Nemaline myopathy (NM) is a group of inherited disorders that affects muscle tone and strength. At various stages in life, the shoulder, upper arm, pelvic and thigh muscles may be affected. Symptoms usually begin between birth and early childhood. There are two main forms of NM:

- Typical: Is the most common form, usually presenting in infants with muscle weakness and floppiness. It may be slowly progressive or non-progressive, and most adults are able to walk.

- Severe: Is characterized by absence of spontaneous movement or respiration at birth, and is often fatal in the first few months of life. Occasionally, late-childhood or adult-onset can occur.

NM is considered rare, affecting approximately 1 in 50,000 people. NM can be caused by a mutation in one of several different genes responsible for making muscle protein.

Symptoms vary depending on the age of onset and the type of NM. They may include:

- Poor muscle tone and weakness (especially in the face, neck, upper arms and legs),

- Delay or inability to walk,

- Breathing problems,

- Difficulty feeding and swallowing,

- Speech difficulties.

Oropharyngeal Muscular Dystrophy

Oculopharyngeal muscular dystrophy (OPMD) is an inherited, adult-onset form of muscular dystrophy that, while found worldwide, affects French Canadian and Jewish populations more frequently. The estimated prevalence in the French-Canadian population of Quebec is 1 in 1,000 people.

OPMD is caused by a mutation in the PABPN1 gene.

Symptoms may include:

- Difficulty swallowing (dysphagia),

- Tongue weakness and atrophy,

- Weakness in the proximal muscles,

- Drooping eyelids (ptosis),

- Difficulty gazing upwards and double vision (diplopia).

Treatment may include:

- Surgery,

- Speech and occupational therapy.

Pompe Disease

Pompe disease is a rare, inherited neuromuscular disorder that causes progressive muscle weakness and loss of muscle tissue.

Pompe disease goes by many different names:

- Acid alpha-glucosidase deficiency,

- Acid Maltase Deficiency (AGM),

- Glycogen Storage Disease Type 2,

- Lysosomal alpha-glucosidase deficiency.

Pompe disease can occur between infancy and adulthood, and affects both men and women equally. Approximately one-third of people with Pompe disease are infants (infantile-onset) while the other two thirds are children or adults (late-onset).

Pompe disease is caused by mutations in a gene that makes an enzyme called acid alpha-glucosidase (GAA). The job of this enzyme is to break down glycogen, a form of sugar stored in muscle cells throughout the body. In people with Pompe disease, this enzyme is either missing or in short supply.

The symptoms and severity of Pompe disease can vary widely from person to person. Symptoms associated with the infantile-onset form may include:

- Feeding and breathing difficulties,

- An enlarged heart, tongue, and liver,

- Inability to gain weight,

- A "frog-like" leg position,

- Breathing problems and frequent respiratory infections.

Symptoms associated with the late-onset form may include:

- Chewing and swallowing difficulties,

- Lower back pain,

- Scoliosis,

- Frequent falls.

Enzyme replacement therapy (ERT) has the ability to treat the underlying cause of the disease. Though ERT is not a cure, providing the missing enzyme may slow the progression of muscle weakness and improve muscle function. Treatment options also include supportive care, such as:

- Respiratory therapies and ventilator assistance,

- Physical therapy,

- Occupational therapy.

Speak with your health care provider about treatment options that are right for you.

Spinal Muscular Atrophy

Spinal muscular atrophy (SMA) is a group of inherited genetic muscle-wasting disorders. SMA affects the nerve cells that control voluntary muscle. These nerve cells are called motor neurons, and SMA causes them to die off. People with SMA are generally grouped into one of four types (I, II, III, IV) based on their highest level of motor function or ability.

- Type I (severe) – also known as infantile-onset or Werdnig-Hoffman disease,

- Type II (intermediate),

- Type III (mild) – also known as Kugelberg-Welander disease,

- Type IV – also known as adult SMA.

SMA is rare condition, occurring in approximately 1 out of every 6,000 live births. It is a autosomal recessive genetic disease. About 1 out of 40 people are genetic carriers of the disease (meaning that they carry the mutated gene but do not have SMA).

SMA is caused by a missing or abnormal (mutated) gene known as survival motor neuron gene 1 (SMN1). In a healthy person, this gene produces a protein in the body called survival motor neuron (SMN) protein. In a person with mutated genes, this protein is absent or significantly decreased, and causes severe problems for motor neurons. Motor neurons are nerve cells in the spinal cord which send out nerve fibers to muscles throughout the body. Since SMN protein is critical to the survival and health of motor neurons, nerve cells may shrink and eventually die without this protein, resulting in muscle weakness.

Neuromuscular Medicine

Neuromuscular medicine includes the diagnosis and treatment of abnormalities of the motor neuron, nerve root, peripheral nerves, neuromuscular junction, and muscle, including disorders that affect adults and children.

The neuromuscular medicine, and physiatry specialists are key health care providers who work cooperatively with a multidisciplinary team to provide coordinated care for persons with Neuromuscular diseases (NMDs). The director or coordinator of the team must be aware of the potential issues specific to NMDs and be able to access the interventions that are the foundations for proper care in NMD. These include health maintenance and proper monitoring of disease progression and complications to provide anticipatory, preventive care and optimum management. Ultimate goals include maximizing health and functional capacities, performing medical monitoring and surveillance to inhibit and prevent complications, and promoting access and full integration into the community in order to optimize quality of life.

The estimated total prevalence of the most common neuromuscular diseases (NMDs) in the United States is 500,000. Combined with all forms of acquired NMDs the prevalence exceeds 4 million which is an impressive figure when compared for example to the prevalence of spinal cord injury, estimated to be between 239,000 to 306,000. There is tremendous diversity of etiologies for both acquired and hereditary neuromuscular diseases. Some NMDs are acquired with diverse causes distinct from genetic etiologies such as autoimmune, infectious, metabolic, toxic, or paraneoplastic (e.g. amyotrophic lateral sclerosis (ALS), myasthenia gravis, lambert eaton syndrome, botulism, Guillain Barre syndrome, or diabetic peripheral neuropathy). There are over 500 distinct NMDs identified to date which have specific genes that have been linked causally to these conditions. Limb girdle muscular dystrophy, for example, has over 20 genetically distinct subtypes that have been identified to date. The genetic heterogeneity of hereditary neuromuscular diseases has created challenges for clinicians and researchers.

Although currently incurable, NMDs are not untreatable. The neuromuscular medicine, and physiatry specialists are key health care providers who work cooperatively with a multidisciplinary team to maximize health, maximize functional capacities (including mobility, transfer skills, upper limb function, and self-care skills), inhibit or prevent complications (such as disuses weakness, skeletal deformities, disuses weakness, airway clearance problems, respiratory failure, cardiac insufficiency and dysrhythmias, bone health problems, excessive weight gain or weight loss, metabolic syndrome), and promote access to full integration into the community with optimal quality of life.

The molecular basis of hereditary NMDs has been emerging and coming into sharper focus over the past three decades. Many promising therapeutic strategies have since been developed in animal models. Human trials of these strategies have started, leading to the hope of definitive treatments for many of these currently incurable diseases. Although specific treatments for NMD have not yet reached the clinic, the natural history of these diseases can be changed by the targeting of interventions to known manifestations and complications. Diagnosis can be swiftly reached; the family and patient can be well supported, and individuals who have NMD can reach their full potential in education and employment. In Duchenne muscular dystrophy for example, corticosteroid, respiratory, cardiac, orthopaedic, and rehabilitative interventions have led to improvements in function, quality of life, health, and longevity, with children who are diagnosed today having the possibility of a life expectancy into their fourth decade.

The comprehensive management of all of the varied clinical problems associated with NMDs is a complex task. For this reason, the interdisciplinary approach is critical. It takes advantage of the expertise of many clinicians, rather than placing the burden on one. This interdisciplinary approach to caring for patients with NMD, and participation by committed providers that have NMD disease-specific expertise are key ingredients to the provision of optimal care. The patient and family / care providers should actively engage with the medical professional who coordinates clinical care. Depending on the patient's circumstances, such as area/country of residence or insurance status, this role might be served by, but is not limited to, a neurologist or pediatric neurologist, physiatrist / rehabilitation specialist, neurogeneticist, pediatric orthopedist, pediatrician, or primary-care physician. In the U.S. the coordination of care is often done by the Neuromuscular Medicine specialist (ACGME approved fellowships in Neuromuscular Medicine now exist for subspecialty certification within the American Board of Psychiatry and Neurology and the American Board of Physical Medicine and rehabilitation). The director or coordinator of the team must be aware of the potential issues specific to NMDs and be able to access the interventions that are the foundations for proper care in NMD. These include health maintenance and proper monitoring of disease progression and complications to provide anticipatory, preventive care and optimum management.

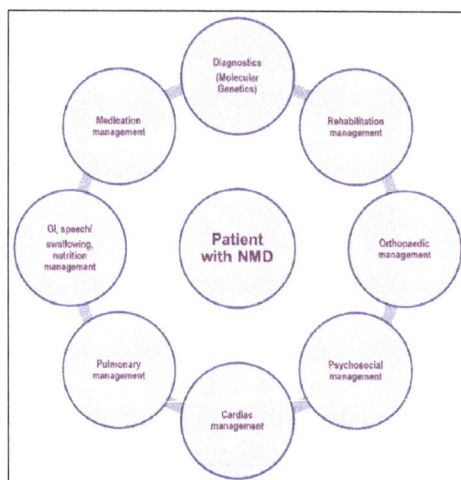

Interdisciplinary NMD Clinical Care Coordination.

Toolkits of Assessments and Interventions

There are varied toolkits of assessments and interventions applicable to NMD management. Input from different specialties and the specific assessments, and interventions will change as the NMD progresses. Some measures such as strength assessment, functional grading, timed function measures, and pulmonary function measures are core measures performed at least annually for most NMDs. Others are performed regularly depending on the expected impairments for specific NMDs.

Selected Assessments for NMD

There are diverse assessments that are performed in NMDs for clinical studies, natural history studies, and clinical trials. Some core measures such as manual muscle testing for strength, ROM, timed function, pulmonary function, and selected cardiac measures are routinely performed annually or more frequently if clinically indicated.

Important clinical data that should be obtained initially on each patient include: gender, birth date, family history, date of disease (symptom) onset, disease duration, dominant limb, weight and height, cardiovascular and pulmonary symptoms and findings, presence of contractures and spine deformity, muscle strength, ambulatory status (including age at cessation of ambulation and years of wheelchair use), and any treatment interventions. When relevant, these data should be updated at each patient visit. In large clinics data can be recorded on a standardized form and entered into a computer database or electronic health record. Records of respiratory and cardiovascular symptoms and findings should be maintained at each clinic visit. The history should include questions relating to shortness of breath with ambulation, at rest, and during sleep; palpitations; dyspnea; and chest pain. A thorough systems study should be made of cardiopulmonary complications, including pneumonia, prolonged upper respiratory tract infections, respiratory compromise requiring assisted ventilation, and heart failure.

Strength Assessments

Precise measures of strength are important for evaluating clinical progression in NMD as well as assessing the efficacy of any interventions. Strength traditionally has been assessed with manual muscle testing (MMT) using the Medical Research Council (MRC) scale for muscle grading, although this is not reliable in muscles that are only mildly affected. Care must be exercised for consistent inter-examiner measures of the anti-gravity muscles.

MRC Grade Degree of Strength:

- 5: Normal strength.

- 5–: Barely detectable weakness.

- 4S: Same as 4 but stronger than reference muscle.

- 4: Muscle is weak but moves the joint against a combination of gravity and some resistance.

- 4W: Same as 4, but weaker than reference muscle.

- 3+: The muscle is capable of transient resistance but collapses abruptly. This degree of weakness is difficult to put into words, but it is a muscle that is able to move the joint against gravity and an additional small amount of resistance. It is not to be used for muscles capable of sustained resistance throughout their whole range of movement.

- 3: Muscle cannot move against resistance but moves the joint fully against gravity. With the exception of knee extensors, the joint must be moved through its full mechanical range against gravity. If a patient has contractures that limit movement of the joint, the mechanical range obviously will be to the point at which the contractures cause a significant resistance to the movement.

- 3–: Muscle moves the joint against gravity but not through the full extent of the mechanical range of the joint.

- 2: Muscle moves the joint when gravity is eliminated.

- 1: A flicker of movement is seen or felt in the muscle.

- 0: No movement.

Quantitative strength measurements are somewhat more labor intensive, but provide more sensitive and reproducible information. These include static (isometric) and dynamic (isokinetic) measurements, most often done in selected muscle groups (usually bilateral knee, elbow, shoulder, and neck flexors and extensors) with a force transducer that displays force output through a digital force monitor. Static pinch strength and grip strength also may be measured using a force transducer, and these measurements followed serially at clinic visits. The highest score from three maximal trials usually is recorded. The hand-held dynamometer (HHD) is perhaps the most practical yet reliable way to obtain quantitative strength testing in the clinic. The HHD is a small device equipped with an internal load cell that operates as a force transducer. The HHD is capable of measuring force generated by a subject against the examiner who holds the device firmly against the subject and provides stabilization (counter-resistance). The maximum force is recorded. Although it does not replace formal quantitative strength testing, the HHD has reasonably good reliability in NMD for weaker muscle groups and is a good alternative to MMT.

Dynamic strength may be assessed using an isokinetic dynamometer at a fixed speed (e.g., 30 degrees per second) for both concentric (shortening) and eccentric (lengthening) contractions. Flexors and extensors should be evaluated through a full range of motion. Parameters that can be measured include peak torque, total work, work per repetition, peak torque to body weight ration, joint angle at peak torque, range of motion, and fatigue index (decrement in work performance over the exercise bout).

Range of Motion Assessments

Passive Joint range of motion (PROM measurements) should be done with a standard goniometer following the protocol used by Brooke and colleagues, and Fowler and colleagues. Joints to be evaluated for contractures include elbow and wrist extension, hip adduction for iliotibial band tightness, hip and knee extension, and ankle dorsiflexion. The definition of clinically significant contractures varies according to the joint. In some joints, even as little as a 7° flexion contracture can result in the center of gravity (COG) falling to an unstable plane (e.g., anterior to the hip joint and posterior to the knee center of rotation). Care must be taken to measure the ROM of two-joint muscles in position of function (e.g., ankle ROM measured with the knee fully extended).

Active ROM (AROM) assesses the participant's ability to recruit muscle strength to perform a muscle contraction through an available ROM. Passive ROM (PROM) is first performed by a clinical evaluator to assess the extensibility of muscle, tendons and ligaments passively through a ROM. This is followed by evaluation of AROM. The assessment of ROM must be performed taking into account what PROM is available due to contracture. AROM and PROM are necessary for appropriate biomechanics in activities such as walking and using the upper extremities for functional activities.

Timed Function Tests

The time to rise from the floor from a supine position (in seconds) follows the protocol reported previously by CIDD, UC Davis, and the Cooperative International Neuromuscular Research Group (CINRG). The assessment is performed in all ambulatory study participants who can perform the test. For standing from supine the velocity is calculated as 1 divided by the time to complete the task. Subjects are given 30 to 60 seconds to complete the task. A subject who is unable to complete the task is given a score of 99 and a velocity which approaches zero.

Time to Climb Four Stairs

The time to climb 4 standard stairs follows the protocol by CIDD, UC Davis, and CINRG. The assessment is performed in children age 2 and older. For the total task of climbing 4 standard stairs, velocity was calculated as 1 divided by the time to complete the task. Subjects are given 30 to 60 seconds to complete the task. A subject who is unable to complete the task are given a score of 99 and a velocity which approaches zero.

Time to Walk/Run Ten Meters

The time to walk/run ten meters follows the protocol reported by CIDD, and UC Davis for 30 feet, and CINRG for 10 meters. The assessment is performed in children age 2 and older. Timed function test velocities were calculated as distance divided by completion time. Velocity for the 10 meter walk/run test is determined by dividing distance (10 meters) by the time to complete the task (in seconds). Subjects are given 30 to 60 seconds to complete the task. A subject who is unable to complete the task are given a score of 99 and a velocity which approaches zero. Other Timed function tests. These may include time to stand from a chair, time to propel a manual wheelchair 10 meters or 30 feet, time to put on a T-shirt, and time to cut out a 3' × 3' pre-marked square from a piece of paper with safety scissors.

Six-Minute Walk Test (6MWT)

We have recently modified the ATS version of the six-minute walt test (6MWT) and validated the test as a clinical endpoint for DMD. Subsequently, there has been widespread utilization of this measure and success of the measure as a primary endpoint in multicenter clinical trials. The modified 6MWT utilizes standard video instructions, a safety chaser to assist the subject up in the event of a fall, and constant rather than intermittent encouragement. Subjects walk around two cones placed 25 meters apart. For the CINRG DMD natural history study, the 6MWT is performed in all participants who can be expected to walk at least 75 meters. A subject who is unable to ambulate 10 meters on a 10 meter walk/run test is given a "0" value for the 6MWT. Using this protocol, we determined the 6MWT to be reliable and valid in DMD at a single center. The primary variable derived from the 6MWT is the six-minute walk distance (6MWD) in meters. For clinical trials where subjects are tested serially, lower values of 6MWD can be obtained in more marginal ambulators. To account for maturational influences we have described the use of age- and height- based percent predicted values for 6MWT. For the DMD subjects we also measure the number of steps taken during the 6MWT with a tally counter or with a step-watch activity monitor placed on the right ankle. This allows the calculation of average stride length and cadence. The 6MWT takes approximately 15 minutes to complete.

9-Hole Peg Test (9-HPT)

The 9-HPT is commercially available, easy and quick to administer, portable test that is used to measure upper limb function and dexterity. The 9-HPT records the time to pick up 9 pegs from a container, put into the holes, and then returned to the container. The test has been validated in all age groups and has high inter-rater and test-retest validity. The 9-HPT shows concurrent and convergent validity, and the measure appears sensitive to change in adults with neuromuscular and musculoskeletal disorders. Both adult and pediatric norms are available. It has been chosen by the NIH Toolbox as a measure of dexterity because it is a very viable tool for longitudinal epidemiologic studies and intervention trials. The primary variable derived from the 9-HPT is completion time in seconds. Total time for administration of the 9-HPT is 10 minutes or less.

Disease-Specific Functional Rating Scales

Disease specific functional rating systems exist for many NMDs. For example, the ALS Functional Rating scale (ALSFRS) is commonly obtained in ALS patients. In DMD, Functional classifications utilize the upper extremity scale reported by Brooke and the lower extremity scales used by Vignos.

ALS Functional Rating Scale-Revised (ALSFRS-R)

The ALSFRS-R assesses patients' levels of self-sufficiency in areas of feeding, grooming, ambulation, communication, and respiratory. The assessment determines the degree of impairment in ALS patients' abilities to function independently in activities of daily living, locomotion, communication, and breathing. It consists of 12 items to evaluate bulbar function, motor function and respiratory function and each item is scored from 0 (unable) to 4 (normal). The ALSFRS has been validated both cross-sectionally and longitudinally against muscle strength testing, the Schwab and England ADL rating scale, the Clinical Global Impression of Change (CGIC) scale, and independent assessments of patient's functional status. The ALSFRS-R is an attractive primary outcome measure in clinical trials of ALS because it is validated, easy to administer, minimizes dropout, reduces cost, and correlates with survival. Unlike the other standard outcome measures currently employed, the ALSFRS-R is also a measure of global function.

Vignos Lower Extremity Functional Grade

The following functional grade was originally described by Vignos; 1: walks and climbs stairs without assistance; 2: walks and climbs stairs with the aid of a railing; 3: walks and climbs stairs slowly with the aid of a railing (over 12 seconds for 4 standard stairs); 4: walks unassisted and rises from chair but cannot climb stairs; 5: walks unassisted but cannot rise from chair or climb stairs; 6: walks only with the assistance or walks independently with long leg braces; 7: walks in long leg braces but requires assistance for balance; 8: Stands in long leg braces but unable to walk even with assistance; 9: is in a wheelchair; 10: is confined to bed.

Brooke Upper Extremity Functional Grade

The following functional grade was originally described by Brooke: 1: Starting with arms at the sides, the patient can abduct the arms in a full circleuntil they touch above the head; 2: Can raise arms above the head only by flexing the elbow; (i.e. shortening the circumference of the movement or using) or using accessory muscles; 3) Cannot raise hands above head but can raise an 8 ounce glass of water to mouth using both hands if necessary; 4: Can raise hands to mouth but cannot raise an 8-ounce glass of water to mouth; 5: Cannot raise hands to mouth but can use hands to hold pen or pick up pennies from the table; 6: Cannot raise hans to mouth and has no useful function of hands. As an optional measure if the patient has a Brooke Grade of 1 or 2 measured by the therapist, it is determined how many Kg of weight can be placed on a shelf above eye level, using one hand.

North Star Ambulatory Assessment (NSAA)

The NSAA is a clinician rated 17-item functional scale designed for ambulant boys with DMD who are able to stand. This evaluation tool assesses functional activities including standing, getting up from the floor, negotiating steps, hopping, and running. The assessment is based on a 3 point rating scale of 2= ability to perform the test normally, 1= Modified method or assistance to perform test, 0=unable to perform the test. Thus, total score can range from 0 (completely non-ambulant) to 34 - no impairment on these assessments. The North Star Ambulatory Assessment is currently also used in several other countries and international clinical trials. NSAA has shown good reliability and validity in multi-center studies as well as good clinical validity through Rasch analysis.

Motor Function Measure (MFM)

The MFM is a recently developed instrument to assess motor function in ambulant and non-ambulant patients with neuromuscular diseases (NMD) aged 6–62 years . The scale is comprised of 32 items, in three dimensions: D1: standing position and transfers (13 items), D2: axial and proximal motor function (12 items), and

D3: distal motor function (7 items). Each test is scored by the therapist on a 4-point Likert scale. Scores for subscales and the composite total score range from 0= worse to 100%= better. In heterogeneous NMD patients, internal consistency, intra- and inter-rater reliability for the global scale and the subscales was excellent, and face validity, convergent validity and discriminant validity were good, Vuillerot showed that the MFM was able to measure changes in motor function over time in DMD and the total score predicted loss of ambulation. The MFM takes 30–40 minutes to complete.

Egen Classification (EK2) Scale

The EK2 scale was developed by the Danish Muscular Dystrophy Association as a clinical tool to assess overall functional ability in non-ambulatory patients with DMD. This tool includes assessments comprised of functional ability measuring upper extremity grade, muscle strength measured with the manual muscle test, and forced vital capacity defined as a percentage of normal values (FVC%). The construct is based on the interaction of physical components such as muscle strength, range of motion, respiratory status, wheelchair dependence and age. The EK scale assesses ten functional categories (EK 1–10), each on a scale of 0=normal to 3= very impaired, contributing to an overall function score of 0 to 30. The EK scale has shown high inter- and intra-rater reliability (ICC-.98) and good construct validity.

Spine Deformity Evaluations

For many NMD patients spine deformity should be evaluated at every clinic visit. Data obtained at the time of the first patient visit and thereafter should include the presence or absence of spine deformity, any interventions, and the patient's age at time of observation. Radiographs should be reviewed and the results for kyphosis and scoliosis recorded along the guidelines recommended by Carman, Fon, and Gupta.

Pulmonary Evaluations

Depending on the specific NMD diagnosis, pulmonary evaluations by a pulmonologist may be indicated. Pulmonary function tests (PFTs) include forced vital capacity (FVC), forced expiratory volume in 1 second (FEV1), FEV1/FVC, maximal voluntary ventilation (MVV), residual volume (RV), peak expiratory flow rate (PEFR), and peak cough flow. Measurements are made using a spirometer (e.g. KoKo spirometer and digidoser, nSpire Health, Inc.) and the pulmonary function data may be interpreted using the Crapo and Polgar normative reference set for 6–7 year old participants or the Hankinson normative reference set for ≥8 year old participants. Maximal inspiratory pressure (MIP) and maximal expiratory pressure (MEP) are helpful and are measured near RV and total lung capacity (TLC), respectively, following the technique described by Black and Hyatt using a direct ready dial gauge force meter and ventilated

T-tube assembly. Three technically satisfactory measurements should be obtained and the maximum reading recorded. Interpretation of MIP and MEP values can be based on Wilson and Domenech-Clar normative pediatric reference sets. Participants are evaluated in a seated position with support for the back and feet and they wear nose clips or have their noses held closed by hand during testing. If necessary, cardboard mouthpiece adapters can be used to enable participants to make a full lip seal. PFTs should be done at least yearly and more frequently if clinical indications exist. If clinically indicated, arterial blood gas studies, pulse oximetry, and/or capnography (CO_2 monitoring) should be obtained. Formal sleep studies may be indicated depending on the NMD diagnosis and results of regular screening studies such as overnight pulse oximetry.

Cardiac Evaluations

Depending on the specific NMD diagnosis, cardiac evaluations by a cardiologists may be indicated. Regular assessments may include ECG, echocardiography, Holter monitoring, and Cardiac: MR Imaging. Standard 12-lead electrocardiograms (ECGs) should be obtained at 1-year intervals. In some diseases, particularly the myopathies with associated cardiomyopathy, echocardiograms are indicated.

Neuropsychological Tests

Neuropsychologic measurements may be helpful in some of these diseases, particularly if there are educational and vocational problems. However, previous reports that used some of the standard measurement tools suggested that subtle physical impairments may have negatively affected the test results. Therefore, caution is advised in interpreting these tests. Tools such as the Category Test, Seashore Rhythm Test, and Speech-Perception Test should be used, if possible, because performance on these instruments is not dependent on motor function.

Patient-Reported Outcomes (PROs)

Consumers, clinical researchers, the Food and Drug Administration, and industry have increasingly recognized the importance of patient-reported outcome (PRO) measures in the determination of clinically meaningful outcomes and validation of clinical and surrogate endpoints for therapeutic trials. There are regulatory requirements that registration studies must incorporate primary endpoints that objectively measure clinically meaningful "life-changing" events with significant impact on health and well-being. In addition, the FDA has strongly recommended inclusion of PRO measures such as health-related quality of life (HRQOL) assessments as an endpoints in all clinical trials. Both global measures of HRQOL and disease-specific NMD measures have been used in NMD populations.

Ongoing Management/Anticipatory Guidance

Once the diagnosis is confirmed, the patient and family should be thoroughly educated about the expected outcome and what problems may be encountered. The Neuromuscular specialist and physiatrist should then assess the patient's and family goals and develop a medical management and rehabilitative program that matches those goals. Palliative care focuses on living well with optimized quality of life despite life expectancy.

Major advances in the understanding of the molecular basis of many NMDs has greatly enhanced diagnostic accuracy and provides the basis for novel therapeutic interventions. There have also been major pharmacologic advances in the treatment of some NMDs, particularly ALS and DMD. The physiatrist may become involved in the prescription of disease-altering medications for the various NMDs, and therefore should familiarize him/herself with the appropriate pharmacologic agents available. In addition, if not directly involved in research, the physiatrist should nonetheless encourage enrollment in experimental protocols, which not only furthers science but provides some hope for the patient. Education and employment are very important with respect to self-esteem, quality of life, and integration into the community and should be emphasized in people with slowly progressive NMD. Patients should be referred to a support group. Support groups often are a great resource, not only for psychologic support but for problem-solving and recycling of equipment.

Given the many advances that have occurred in the management of people with NMD, many patients will survive through their childbearing years, possibly having children, and can expect to enjoy a good quality of life. The physiatrist can play a critical role during important life transitions and provide care which can maximize function and quality of life.

Neuromuscular Diseases and Rehabilitation

Identification and Classification of NMD

Neuromuscular diseases (NMDs) are a heterogeneous group of diseases that are inherited or acquired, resulting from an abnormality in the anterior horn motor cells, peripheral nerves, neuromuscular junctions, or muscles. The most common neuromuscular diseases are motor neuron diseases, neuropathies, neuromuscular junction diseases, and muscular diseases based on anatomic localization.

Motor neuron diseases are a group of diseases that progress with lower and/or upper motor neuron involvement in motor neurons in the anterior horn of medulla spinalis. They are characterized by muscle weakness associated with fasciculation and atrophy that differs with respect to the location and function of the affected motor neurons. Hereditary spinal muscular atrophy (SMA) is the most common motor neuron disease. SMA is caused by the degeneration of the anterior horn cells in the spinal cord and brain stem and by the activation of the corticospinal tract. Progressive symmetrical weakness, hypotonia, hyporeflexia or areflexia, muscle atrophy, fasciculation typically affecting the tongue, and postural tremor in the fingers are typical signs and symptoms of SMA. Spasticity may also be seen as a disease-specific finding in patients with upper motor neuron involvement such as amyotrophic lateral sclerosis (ALS).

Neuropathies are peripheral nerve diseases with sensory and motor symptoms. The observation of sensory changes in addition to muscle weakness distinguishes peripheral nerve diseases from diseases of other components of the motor unit. It causes demyelination in the nerve and axonal degeneration in the nerve by affecting the nerve myelin sheath and/or axon. The most common neuropathies are hereditary, but there are also different syndromes such as inflammatory, toxic, and infectious neuropathies. The loss of muscular strength and muscular atrophy is observed starting from feet and legs in the lower extremity and hands in the upper extremity, while paresthesia/dysesthesia is observed in a stocking-glove distribution. The most common Charcot-Marie-Tooth (CMT) disease or hereditary motor and sensory neuropathy constitutes a genetically heterogeneous group of diseases affecting the peripheral nervous system. CMT, which is characterized by the abnormal development or degeneration of the peripheral nerve, has different genetic pattern transitions. The disease begins during infancy in many cases. Symptoms include inadequate gait, muscular atrophy and weakness progressing from the distal to proximal extremities, foot deformities such as cavus deformity, deep tendon reflex loss, and sensory loss in the distal extremities. Inappropriate gait may be evident as walking with jumping and there may be a prone to falling. Hereditary neuropathies are diseases affecting peripheral nerves and classified as hereditary motor and sensory neuropathies (HMSNs), hereditary motor neuropathies, hereditary sensory neuropathies, and hereditary sensory and autonomic neuropathies. Autonomic neuropathies include loss of sweating, bladder dysfunction, constipation, and impotence in males.

Neuromuscular junction diseases are autoimmune diseases that result from the destruction, impairment, or absence of one or more proteins during neuromuscular transmission. Most neuromuscular junction diseases are acquired and occur associated with presynaptic, synaptic, and postsynaptic disorders. Myasthenia gravis (MG), the result of a postsynaptic disorder, is the most common neuromuscular transmission disorder. MG has two clinical forms: ocular and generalized. Weakness in the ocular form is limited to the eyelids and extraocular muscles. In generalized myasthenic patients, however, there is also a weakness in the bulbar, extremity, and respiratory muscles in varying degrees due to the cranial involvement. As a result, ptosis, diplopia, dysphagia, and dysarthria are observed. Myasthenic weakness typically fluctuates during the day, usually the least in the morning, and worsens as the day progresses with prolonged use of muscles, especially those that are stiff.

The main problem in muscle diseases involves the degeneration in muscle rather than in the nerve. It is a group of genetic diseases proceeding with progressive muscle weakness that causes subsequent limitation of joint movements, shortness of muscles, a decrease in respiratory capacity, and posture disorders. The loss of function in the body and in the upper and lower limb, impairment of organization of postural reactions, fatigue, loss of cardiopulmonary adjustment, and disturbed psychosocial condition are among the clinical and functional problems encountered. Different functional levels and clinical characteristics may be observed ranging from minimal influence to being confined to bed depending on the type of disease, the age of onset, and the location of the affected muscle group (proximal and/or distal). Bed confinement is observed in the early period in Duchenne musculoskeletal dystrophy (DMD) and Becker muscular dystrophy (BMD). However, facioscapulohumeral musculoskeletal dystrophy (FSHMD) and limb-girdle muscular dystrophy (LGMD) progress slowly and decrease the patient's functional ability and quality of life by causing scoliosis, wing scapula, difficulty in going up or down the stairs, toe walking and lordotic posture, difficulty in standing up from a sitting or squatting position, and Gower's sign. Gower's sign indicates the weakness of the proximal muscles, namely those of the lower limb. The sign describes a patient that has to use their hands and arms to "walk" up their own body from a squatting position due to lack of hip and thigh muscle strength, and contractures are observed. In many types of diseases, the decreased pulmonary function is due to the respiratory muscle weakness and spinal deformities (kyphoscoliosis), which leads to respiratory tract infections and respiratory disorders. Cardiomyopathy and arrhythmia lead to cardiac failure and this cardiorespiratory complications cause death. In the literature, various classifications were done according to the rate of progression of the disease, the affected area, and the body part involved, but the most recent classification was done according to the Belgian Neuromuscular Disease Registry.

According to the international classification of health, function, and disability (ICF) by the World Health Organization (WHO), neuromuscular disorders are associated with disability in body structure and function, resulting in problems with activity and participation. These problems in muscle diseases can be addressed in two parts: primary and secondary. Primary disorders are muscular pain, atrophy, pseudohypertrophy, myotonia, and the loss of postural control, while the secondary ones are fatigue, difficulty in transfer activities and mobility problems, exercise intolerance, contractures, respiration, and psychological problems. The problems observed in the patient are related to the type of disease, pathogenesis, and progression of illness.

Table: Classification of neuromuscular diseases.

1. Muscular dystrophies	2. Myotonic and relaxation disorders	3. Myopathies	4. Disorder of the neuromuscular transmission	5. Disorder of the motor neurons	6. Neuropathies
1. Congenital muscular dystrophy2. Duchenne muscular dystrophy3. Becker muscular dystrophy4. Dystrophinopathy5. Facioscapulohumeral dystrophy6. Limb girdle muscular dystrophy7. Emery-Dreifuss muscular dystrophy8. Distal myopathy9. Oculopharyngeal muscular dystrophy10. Myotonic dystrophy type 111. Myotonic dystrophy type 212. Other muscular dystrophies	1. Thomsen-type myotonia congenita2. Becker-type myotonia congenita3. Paramyotonia congenita4. Familial periodic paralysis5. Other myotonic disorders	a. Congenital myopathies1. Central core disease2. Multiminicore disease3. Nemaline myopathy4. Myotubularb. Myopathy5. Centronuclear myopathy6. Fiber-type disproportion myopathy7. Metabolic myopathies8. Muscle glycogenoses9. Disorders of fatty acid metabolism mitochondrial myopathyc. Inflammatory myopathies10. Polymyositis11. Dermatomyositis12. Inclusion body myositis13. Other myopathies	1. Myasthenia gravis2. Congenital myasthenia3. Lambert-Eaton syndrome4. Other disorders of neuromuscular transmission	1. Amyotrophic lateral sclerosis2. Primary muscular atrophy3. Postpolio syndrome4. Primary lateral sclerosis5. Werdnig-Hoffman spinal muscular atrophy6. Intermediate spinal muscular atrophy7. Kugelberg-Welander spinal muscular atrophy8. Adult spinal muscular atrophy9. X-linked bulbo-spinal muscular atrophy or Kennedy's disease10. Distal spinal muscular atrophy11. Hereditary spastic paraplegia12. Other disorders of motor neurons	a. Hereditary1. Hereditary motor and sensory neuropathy2. Hereditary neuropathy with liability to pressure palsies3. Hereditary sensory & autonomous neuropathyb. Inflammatory4. Guillain-Barré syndrome5. Chronic inflammatory demyelinating polyneuropathy6. Multifocal motor neuropathy7. Vasculitis8. Neuropathy associated with paraproteinemia9. Neuropathy associated with plasma cell dyscrasia10. Amyloisdosis11. Neuropathy in systemic disease12. Other neuropathies
					7. Hereditary ataxias and others

Body Structure and Function Disorders in NMD according to the International Classification of Function

Loss of Strength

The progressive loss of strength, severity of which changes depending on the type of the disease, is one of the leading problems that constitute the deficiencies seen in neuromuscular diseases. The functional deficiencies seen in neuromuscular diseases vary depending on the localization of affected muscle groups and secondary outcomes caused by muscle weakness vary depending on the type and progression of the disease but it should be remembered that the severity of the disease may vary due to the individual differences among the patients. The loss of strength can be seen in the distal and/or proximal region. Also, the loss of strength can also be seen in the neck and mimic muscles. The reason for the progressive loss of muscle strength in neuromuscular diseases varies according to the nature of the disease. It is due to the reduction in the number and size of intrinsic contractile fibers in muscle diseases that are followed by replacement of these fibers by fat infiltration and connective tissue. These changes are caused by the disturbance in the nerve stimulation and transmission pathways necessary for muscle contraction. Also, the decrease in the optimal length of the muscle and deterioration of the sarcomere structure resulting from decreased physical activity secondary to the disease is among the causes of the development of immobilization. It has been shown in the literature that the muscle ceasing to the contraction has lost half of its strength after 3–5 weeks. For example, patients with FSMD typically show weakness around the shoulder and facial muscles, thereby weakening the activities involving the upper extremity for function, while DMD typically shows weakness around the hips of the patients. Thus, patients have difficulty in activities involving the lower extremities. Approximately 75% of muscle patients have muscle strength loss in the proximal limb of the extremity, 20% in the facioscapulohumeral, and 4% in the scapuloperoneal part of the body. However, in acquired diseases (such as inflammatory myopathy), a loss of strength occurs subacutely. Some neuromuscular diseases affect specific muscles. FSHMD should be considered if there is asymmetric loss of strength in the muscles around the scapula, humerus, facial, and mimic muscles. Myotonic dystrophy (MD) should primarily be considered if there is involvement of the frontal and facial muscles, as well as the sternocleidomastoid muscle and the distal (especially tibialis anterior) muscles.

In CMT disease, in which foot and ankle problems and especially muscle weakness are commonly seen, weakness typically begins in the intrinsic muscles of the foot and follows the peroneus brevis and longus, tibialis anterior, extensor digitorum longus, and extensor hallucis longus muscles. This weakness pattern causes the muscle imbalance; while the plantar flexors remain relatively strong, the dorsiflexors weaken and consequently leads to the contraction of the Achilles tendon. As a secondary to this muscle imbalance, together with calcaneus inversion, forefoot adduction, and claw toe, pes cavus deformity develops typically in CMT disease. Also, symptoms such as drop head, ptosis, dysphagia, and dysarthria can be seen in oculopharyngeal muscular dystrophy. In patients with peripheral neuropathy, however, the loss of muscle strength has been shown to be more prominent in the foot dorsiflexors, knee extensors, and hip flexor muscles.

Postural Control and Balance Problems

The strength necessary for the movement of the extremities is generated, collected, and transferred to the upper extremity from the lower extremity by the postural control. Thus, the segments from the proximal to distal that are independent of each other operate in a specific interaction and concordance during functional activities.

The efferent system is composed of the structures necessary for postural control including vestibular, visual, and somatosensory inputs. The somatosensory input disorders can disrupt the postural control and lead to falls in neuromuscular diseases, which causes various conditions such as the weakness of the proximal or distal extremity (like patients with myopathy), axial weakness (myositis or amyotrophic lateral sclerosis), stiffness (myotonia), slow muscle contraction (nemaline myopathy), intermittently varying weakness (myasthenia gravis), sensory polyneuropathic end-effector proprioceptive (myasthenia gravis), and sensory polyneuropathy resulting in proprioceptive insufficiency. While the efferent system is also necessary to maintain a similar upright stabilization, it provides effective postural correction after perturbations during posture. The inadequacy of the efferent system can disrupt balance control and cause falls.

One of the problems that threaten postural control in neuromuscular diseases is the progressive nature of muscle weakness; the other is the inactivity due to the loss of ambulation following the progression. In both cases, spinal stabilization is affected due to the motor and postural reasons, leading to spinal problems. In cases where the ambulation continues despite the decrease in muscular strength, many postural problems such as lordosis, kyphosis, scoliosis, and wing scapula are observed due to the increase in the compensatory responses in the body.

Scoliosis develops before the loss of ability to walk in 30% of muscle patients. The restriction of the paraspinal muscles causing the lordotic sitting posture in extension emerges as a result of locking of the posterior facets of the vertebral bone and the vertebral bones remaining flattened. In addition, kyphotic sitting position is also preferred by patients as a result of the weakened paraspinal muscles. This kyphotic position prevents the locking of the posterior facets of the vertebral bones and causes the opening of the joint faces, vertebral rotation, and lateral curve formation. Finally, the functional scoliosis develops as a result of the inability of the vertebrae to resist to the gravity, the multifaceted adverse influencing of the posture, and difficulty in controlling this effect.

One of the major problems in the clinical postural control is pelvic obliquity. It affects the sitting balance and causes increased pressure on the lower ischial tuberosity, making the sitting position uncomfortable. Also, the hip joint left on the higher side in the pelvic obliquity tends to be subluxated. Subluxation of the hips may also be observed secondary to progressive muscle weakness. The increasing pelvic obliquity affects spinal stabilization. This condition affects the sitting balance of the patients and causes complaints of pain.

Hip movements are an important factor in correcting lateral balance; hence, proximal muscle weakness can disrupt the ability to balance during external shocks. Distal muscle weakness can lead to falls through different ways; the obstacles that do not look dangerous in normal barrier-free environments can cause the patients with dropped foot to stumble and lose balance, increasing the risk of falls. In studies, it is emphasized that the rotations and movements of the ankles during standing is essential for maintaining and correcting the balance.

The wing scapula is observed in patients due to power loss in the shoulder girdle. Wing scapula adversely affects upper extremity functions. Kyphosis and dropped head syndrome have been reported in some myopathies, particularly due to loss of strength in the neck extensor muscles. Patients with dropped head syndrome experience severe walking difficulty with loss of spinal smoothness.

Proprioception plays an important role in stabilizing the body during both comfortable posture and unexpected postural perturbations. Therefore, patients with peripheral neuropathy are unstable when their eyes are closed during standing. In addition, reflex responses to postural perturbations are either delayed or decreased in amplitude or both.

In addition to the above-mentioned findings that are directly related to postural control, postural control plays an important role in many activities such as stair climbing, wheelchair activities, writing, bathing, makeup, shaving, eating, toilet needs, and in-bed mobility.

Atrophy

In this disease group that proceeds with progressive muscle weakness, the patients become more inactive and sedentary in time because the muscles are the active structures responsible for movement in the body. It is stated in the literature that atrophy develops between 14 and 17% of muscle fiber after 72 h of immobilization. Atrophy in muscular diseases develops later compared to peripheral nerve diseases. Selective atrophy of certain muscles may be associated with disease-specific disorders.

Pseudohypertrophy

Pseudohypertrophy is a false hypertrophy seen in the muscle. The hypertrophic appearance of fibrils in the affected muscles results from the replacement of the fibrils by the fat and connective tissue. It does not cause a real increase in the strength of the muscle even though the muscle volume increases. The hypertrophy in the muscle fibers that have not yet been lost is accompanied by the increase in the fat and connective tissue, and thus muscle mass increases. It is most commonly seen in the gastrocnemius-soleus muscle group, occasionally in quadriceps, biceps brachii, and deltoid muscles. In addition, the presence of atrophic muscles around the muscles of the pseudohypertrophy may exaggerate this enlarged image.

Myotonia

Clinically, myotonia refers to any condition that prevents the relaxation of the muscles after contraction. The relaxation difficulty is evident in the first movement of the muscle after its resting position. Relaxation difficulty is reduced when the same movement is repeated after which the movements become easier. Although this is the only symptom in some diseases, in myotonic dystrophy it is associated with permanent muscle strength loss. Myotonia seen in MD and ALS is a factor affecting patients' lives negatively in activities such as handshaking and jar opening.

Pain

Pain is an important problem in most of NMDs, but it is not typically a direct consequence of disease, and now researchers agree that chronic pain is a common symptom that can be seen in all forms of NMDs. In a study on 511 NMPs involving DMD, BMD (myotonic musculoskeletal dystrophy (MMD), metabolic myopathy, FSHMD, and MG), Guy-Coichard et al. evaluated the frequency, characteristics, and effects of pain; they found that the pain was moderate to severe in NMDs and emphasized that pain should be regularly assessed in this patient group. Pain observed in neuromuscular diseases is the result of progressive muscle weakness, fatigue, ligament laxity or stretching, and abnormality of walking and posture. In neuropathic conditions, however, pain-causing mechanisms are neurogenic inflammation, abnormal involvement of the sympathetic nervous system, and the neuroplasticity changes in the central nervous system. In a study aiming to determine the structure and location of pain in muscle patients, 73% of the patients complained of pain, and 27% of them were found to have severe pain. In another study involving the evaluation of pain in 125 patients with neuromuscular disease from different groups, 73% complained of pain, 62% had chronic pain, and 15% had severe pain. The localization of the pain was reported to be spinal column in 81%, shoulder girdle in 54%, hip in 47%, and knee in 47%. In addition, 67% of these patients reported an increase in pain with walking and 68% with standing.

Contracture

Joint contractures, subluxations, and dislocations are common problems in NMDs. When the strength of the muscles around the same joint is different from each other, the joint tends to remain at a certain position, the corresponding muscle becomes shortened, and this position of the joint is fixed in time, resulting in the formation of contracture. The development of contracture occurs in patients with NMDs in time. The stiffness, which develops in the tendon and increases until contracture occurs, can be prevented or reduced by exercise or splints holding the joint in the opposite position.

Flexion contracture is seen in hip joint with loss of strength of the hip extensor. The lumbar lordosis is increased so that the upright posture can be sustained and the loss of strength can be compensated. However, the progression of the weakness in the muscles of the pelvic girdle causes the knee flexion contracture to develop. The increasingly apparent loss of strength in the gluteus maximus and quadriceps muscle leads to an excessively increased lordosis. As the patient tries to stabilize hips in the extension, lordosis becomes more pronounced. As the muscles weaken, the patient tries to increase stabilization by pulling the arms back and increasing the lordosis to pull the center of gravity behind the hip joint. Due to the loss of dorsiflexor muscle strength, plantar flexion contracture develops in the ankle joint, resulting in toe walking.

Cardiopulmonary Problems

Neuromuscular diseases cause respiratory problems mainly due to the inadequacy of the respiratory muscles, namely upper airway muscles (mouth and tongue muscles), external intercostal muscles, diaphragm, and abdominal muscles. The restrictive type of respiratory problem is observed in particular. Along with the involvement of the primary respiratory muscles in Becker MD and FSHMD, respiratory problems are encountered. The compliance of the chest wall is reduced, and then, there becomes a decrease in the total lung capacity. The disease may also cause kyphoscoliosis that increases the respiratory problem. Muscle fatigue in MG bears respiratory problems, whereas bulbar involvement in ALS causes increased secretion, inability to close glottis, and decreased respiratory control. In MM dystrophy and congenital myotonic dystrophy, a direct cardiac involvement is in the form of cardiomyopathies observed in addition to respiratory problems. Respiratory disturbances and cardiomyopathy may follow the development of scoliosis. Respiratory muscle strength is insufficient in muscle patients. In particular, the maximal inspiratory (MIP) and expiratory (MEP) pressures are below normal values.

The respiratory muscle weakness that emerges in the late stages of any neuromuscular disease results in hypoventilation and hypercapnia. This causes restrictive pulmonary impairment and reduced exercise capacity. Moreover, during terminal stages of all diseases with muscle involvement, the weakness in the respiratory muscles restricts coughing. This problem may result in difficulty in swallowing and aspiration pneumonia. This in turn may cause the mechanical ventilator to be connected. While cardiac involvement is mostly a result of respiratory involvement, it can be primarily seen as cardiac muscle involvement in some NMDs. In patients whose heart muscle is affected, the heart will have difficulty adapting to changes in the body in the event of any increase in physical activity.

The presence of cardiomyopathy resulting from a lack of dystrophin in the myocardium and cardiac Purkinje fibers affects the cardiopulmonary response to exercise. Myocardial dysfunction remains silent due to decreased physical activity until the end of the disease process. The effect of cardiomyopathy and restrictive pulmonary disease on physical activity is much greater in NMDs with slower progression.

Activity Problems in NMD

Although most neuromuscular disorders have progressive and clinically distinct features, the most important common feature is that they lead to functional problems and activity limitations at various levels. The activity limitations due to the functional deficits vary depending on the localization of the affected region, on the type of the disease with secondary outcomes caused by loss of strength, and even on the patient. The patients with muscle diseases usually go to the doctor with complaints such as difficulty in climbing stairs or a slope, getting up from the sitting position, walking, raising arms and reaching up, and washing the head. The patients may also complain about numbness in feet and hands and not being able to open eyes, and difficulty in swallowing. At the end of the natural progression of the disease, there may be a loss of strength in both the proximal and distal muscles and the inability to perform many activities such as wheelchair activities, writing, bathing, applying makeup, shaving, eating, toilet needs, and mobility within the bed.

Fatigue, cardiopulmonary effect, and exercise intolerance cause an increase in fat mass and contractures. It also causes a decrease in the efficient use of locomotion (such as reduced walking space and more energy expenditure), a decreased motivation of the patient, a reduction in support of the social environment for activity, an increase in depression, and social barriers. These restrictions all result in a decline in physical activity performance in NMDs. The progressive muscle weakness present in NMD directly affects the daily activities of the patient. Depending on the degree of muscle weakness in the proximal part of the body, patients may have difficulty in fine hand skills such as self-care, dressing, and hygiene. The patients may also have difficulty in transfers requiring upper extremity support, ambulation activities, reaching to mouth due to the weakness of the distal muscle groups, bilateral use of cutlery, and nail clipping. In a study involving 208 neuromuscular patients, Pieterse have grouped the activities that the patients had difficulty under the following headings: (1) communication, (2) eating and drinking, (3) transfer, (4) walking and moving around, (5) transportation, (6) lifting and carrying, (7) fine hand skill, and (8) use of arms higher than shoulder level.

Fatigue

More than 60% of patients with NMD complain about severe fatigue along with muscle weakness and many other problems. Fatigue has a significant effect on exercise limitation and includes the physiological fatigue and the experienced fatigue. The physiological fatigue is defined as an exercise-dependent reduction in maximal voluntary muscle strength while the experienced fatigue is defined as difficulty in initiation and maintenance of voluntary activities. The physiological fatigue is the one with both peripheral and central components, either muscular or related to limitation initiated in the central nervous system (CNS). Many mechanisms may cause this fatigue and exercise limitation. In neuromuscular diseases, there is the fatigue (peripheral fatigue) stemming from the local effects on the muscle function on one side, and there is the fatigue (central fatigue) arising from the level of CNS due to the feedback of the pathological condition in the peripheral nervous system on the other side. This type of fatigue protects the muscle from being damaged in the long term during the improperly set physical activities. This symptom is perceived by patients as a different, abnormal, and feeling of being more tired than before the onset of disease. In a study, which included the neuromuscular disease groups of HMSN, FSHMD, and MG, is indicated that severe fatigue is associated with functional impairment in daily life. The level of fatigue has been found to be significantly related to the muscular strength, the level of physical activity stated by the patient, sleep disorders, and pain. The fatigue level and the physical activity level are mostly associated with functional impairment in daily life.

Exercise Intolerance and the Impact on Functional Capacity

Exercise intolerance is a type of abnormally severe tiredness that develops with a certain movement in the muscle involved in that movement. In individuals with NMHD, several factors such as loss of functional muscle tissue, unused muscles, injuries due to excessive use, cardiopulmonary involvement, contractures, decreased locomotion adequacy (decreased walking speed and increased energy expenditure), decreased patient motivation, less social participation for activity, increased depression, and increased social barriers lead to a decline in physical activity. Three problems affecting functional capacity and determining the level of physical activity in NMD are often striking. These are muscle weakness, difficulty in exercising, and fatigue. These problems result in a decrease in physical activity and a sedentary lifestyle. Unfortunately, sedentary behavior increases exercise intolerance and causes a decrease in functional capacity in the subsequent periods, resulting in a low quality of life. The occurrence of fatigue is dependent on which of the energy-producing metabolic pathways were used during the activity. For example, if a patient develops exercise intolerance while walking but this patient is not uncomfortable while running fast, this should primarily suggest the impairment of lipid metabolism, which enables slow movements with type-1 muscle fibers. On the other hand, if the same complaint occurs in the arm muscles, for example, in an arm movement such as serial and rapid wiping, it should be primarily considered that the glycogen metabolism used by the type-2 muscle fibers is defective in this case. Individuals who have been diagnosed with NMD are more likely to live a sedentary life when compared to physically healthy people. A person with a lower level of physical activity will later have an increased body weight even with a normal diet. Increased body weight makes the patient more inactive, and this continues in a vicious cycle. Therefore, when it is considered that all of the components required for exercise are relatively affected in NMDs, a reduction in exercise capacity in this disease group is inevitable.

Walking and Mobility Problems

Mobility is defined as the movement of the person around self and transition from one position to another in a safe manner; it is a function that should be carefully observed throughout the course of the disease in NMD. NMDs progress with disorders limiting the patients' mobility and their independence in daily life activities. The reason for this is that the progressive weakness of the muscles affects the functional levels of the patients negatively after a while, leading to the defects in mobility activities such as standing up, walking, running, and stair climbing. In the majority of NMDs, there is a chronic clinical course emerging slowly or progressing with a rapid decline in muscle strength that leads to impaired motor function. Neuromuscular patients suffer from difficulty in standing up from the ground as clinical signs of weakness of hip extensors, quadriceps, and trunk muscles. The increasingly apparent loss of power in the gluteus maximus and quadriceps muscles leads to an excessively increased lordosis. As the patient tries to stabilize hips in extension, lordosis becomes more pronounced. As the muscles weaken, the patient tries to increase stabilization by pulling the arms back and increasing the lordosis to pull the center of gravity behind the hip joint. To expand the area of support while walking, the patient walks like a duck (Trendelenburg gait). Fracture contracture is seen in hip joint with the loss of strength in hip extensor and the lumbar lordosis is increased so that the upright posture can be sustained and the loss of strength can be compensated. However, the progression of the loss of strength in the muscles of the pelvic girth causes the knee flexion contracture to develop. The weakness of the hip flexor and the eccentric muscle reduces the length of stride. The weakness of the knee extensor reduces the knee flexion moment in the midstance phase. Due to the weakness of dorsiflexion, plantar flexion contracture obstructs the stabilization of the foot during standing as well as the toe-off during the swing phase.

Contractures may lead to postural disorders such as kyphoscoliosis and scoliosis, which can interfere with the continuation of sitting and lying activities, and as a result, pain. Furthermore, ortheses that help maintain the force, which reduce the development of contractures and deformities, and surgical medical procedures lead to additional disorders. In the advanced stages of NMDs, various problems are faced such as wheelchair dependence, being confined to bed, difficulty in in-bed transfers, inability to maintain mobility during climbing the stairs without holding to something like railing, not being able to stand up from the sitting position, and falling in and out of home. This makes the patients dependent during their daily life activities.

Psychological and other Problems

Even in normal individuals, being ill affects a person psychologically. In a condition such as that of neuromuscular patients where the disease is chronic and has many symptoms, this can make one feel more vulnerable. While some of the patients may cope with the problems associated with the illness and adapt to the social life, some of them respond to these problems with limitations in school, social life, and daily activities. These restrictions manifest themselves as a decrease in independence and self-confidence, limited participation, and social isolation, particularly in youngsters. For example, of two patients with muscular diseases with the same mobility level and the same severity of pain, one may continue to work while the other may quit or even show severe depression. In patients with NMDs, patients with increasing problems are severely affected, and with symptoms such as pain and fatigue, patients may not maintain their psychological well-being.

Participation Problems in NMD

It has been shown in the literature that mobility (transfers and walking), which is one of the parameters of social participation, housekeeping, community life, education, work, and leisure activities were affected in NMD. Biomechanical problems present in NMDs lead to participation problems as a result of the increased energy expenditure levels and fatigue.

Falling and Fear of Falling

According to ICF, falling affects participation by deterioration of the affected body structure and body functions. Falling often has a complex form; it is defined as lying on the ground or at a lower level by accident, except conscious positional change for resting on seats, walls, or other objects, and is affected by multiple factors. There are different descriptions, such as intrinsic and extrinsic factors, associated with the risk factors of falling. These descriptions include age, duration of illness, presence of prior falls, fear of falling, the number of used medicines, use of antihypertensive medicine, reduction in mobility level, and in-home and out-of-home dangers. Also, risk factors include muscle weakness, the presence of falling history, gait abnormality, balance disorder, the use of assistive device, mobility limitation, visual disturbances, arthritis, depression, cognitive impairment/mental status changes, postural hypotension, vertigo/dizziness, incontinence, and chronic diseases. Prevention and reduction of falling have a positive effect on the patient's activity and participation level.

Environmental Factors

Participation problems are encountered as a result of the interaction of environmental factors experienced. Slippery floors, bed-chair heights, poor lighting, unsuitable ancillary equipment, improper building designs, and broken or uneven pavements may be listed among the factors.

Psychological Factors

As the disabilities and difficulties start to be permanent in a patient's life, the patient may lose hope completely. Such people remove themselves from activities and social life, and face many problems including depression as a consequence. Hopelessness, the thought that no one can help them, is a common feeling for neuromuscular patients. In a study of 88 male patients with progressive musculoskeletal dystrophy, it was found that patients had problems in participating in private life and professional life and that more than half of the cases considered themselves to be socially isolated. In his work to assess participation in myotonic dystrophies, Gagnon noted that the participation problems of these patients were about communication, personal care, and interpersonal relationships.

In NMD, the restriction of participation occurs in professional life, leisure activities, home, family, community, and social life. Muscle weakness and reduced aerobic capacity may negatively affect participating in the professional life that requires long-term physical activity. Deterioration of interpersonal interaction and relationships is another reason for the restriction of participation. Sometimes, this restriction can lead to extreme consequences such as no communication with people or not being able to eat or drink in public. Participation in the community and social life can also decrease due to depression and fatigue. The psychological burden of having a degenerative and terminal illness affects the participation of the individual. The presence of each of these factors has significant adverse effects on the quality of life.

Assessment Methods in Rehabilitation of NMD

Nowadays, the key to planning a good rehabilitation program is to know the characteristics of the disease and the problems it will cause in the patient, and to evaluate the patient in detail in light of these features. In NMDs, evaluation is performed to monitor the progression of the disease, to determine the appropriate treatment methods, to investigate the efficacy of treatment methods, and to predict and prevent possible complications. Some evaluation methods are used, in which the disorders of the body structure and function, and the limitations of activity and participation are evaluated. These methods include evaluation of respiratory functions, muscle testing, normal joint movement, evaluation of flexibility, evaluation of motor functions and functional capacities, timed performance tests, functional posture, and gait analysis.

Assessment of Muscle Strength

Due to the diversity of neuromuscular diseases, it is crucial to determine the pattern or spatial distribution of weakness in the evaluation of muscular weakness to distinguish the etiology. It should be determined whether the loss of strength is general (e.g., bilateral, proximal, distal, or all) or localized. The presence of the weakness predominantly in the proximal muscle groups or the dominance in the distal muscles, its presence on one or both sides of the body, and impairment in a single nerve or a group of nerves reflect the pattern of weakness. In the case of huge weakness, it is determined whether the loss of function is proximal or distal, and which functional activities are limited by muscle weakness. If the patient is having difficulty in standing up (around the hips) or combing the hair (around the shoulders), it indicates proximal muscle weakness, commonly observed among the weaknesses in myopathic diseases. If the weakness is pronounced around the hip, there are difficulties in getting up and down the stairs, standing up from the chair or toilet, or standing up from the ground or squatting position. If there is a weakness in the shoulder, there are many functional difficulties such as lifting heavy objects, reaching to and taking the objects on high shelves, brushing teeth, bathing, dressing, and combing the hair. Generally speaking, proximal muscle weakness seen in the form of a limb-girdle pattern in the arms and legs and the muscle group of the shoulder and the hip circumference suggests a myopathic process (process affecting the muscles directly); the presence of distal weakness, however, primarily suggests prevalent polyneuropathy.

However, some myopathies cause distal weakness. This pattern usually cannot be diagnosed and diagnostic errors are possible in relation to the neurogenic feature. The types of myopathic diseases with this atypical distal phenotype are known as distal myopathies and include MD and inclusion body myositis. In less frequent cases of distal myopathies and neuropathies, patients complain of distal upper extremity weaknesses that cause difficulty in activities such as opening jars, buttoning, turning the key, and turning the door handle. Patients with distal lower-limb muscle weakness complain about tripping over the pavement edges, having difficulty walking on uneven surfaces, or dragging feet during walking. Patients experience difficulties standing on toes (m. gastrosoleus) or in activities involving hands (intrinsic muscles).

Methods such as manual muscle testing, dynamometric evaluation, isokinetic (eccentric and concentric) evaluation, and surface electromyography (EMG) are used in the clinical evaluation of muscle strength, but manual muscle test (MMT) is the most commonly used method because of its easy application in clinical practice. Static and isometric contractions of the muscles are also measured with cable tensiometers or dynamometers. These measurements are superior methods because they provide numerical data in NMD, are objective, and reflect changes in muscular strength. However, manual muscle strength measurements remain valid today because of the low reliability of dynamometric measures in muscle groups that cannot complete their movements against the gravity or distal muscle groups. Nevertheless, the physiotherapist who will perform the muscle testing in NMD should be able to analyze whether the factors that limit muscle strength stem from weakness, loss of motor control, pain and/or fatigue, or whether the movements completed during manual muscle testing through compensations. Also, the physiotherapist should consider the time and quality of contraction, the range of motion (ROM) of the joint, and patient's ability to maintain contractions.

For this reason, the evaluating physiotherapist should have performed a significant number of MMT-related applications in neuromuscular diseases. Another method is to find the maximum weight that a person can lift at once. For this purpose, isokinetic instruments have been developed that measure the maximum force at the specified speed in NMDs. These tools give information about both concentric and eccentric contraction. Studies have shown that it is reliable in good unipolar joints, especially elbows and knees. The use of these instruments is somewhat reliable because it is difficult to isolate the shoulder, wrist, and ankle muscles while measuring their strengths during particular movements. It is stated that it is more suitable to perform the force measurement using hand dynamometers providing better stabilization in these joints.

Assessment of Range of Motion and Flexibility

Since there is the loss of muscle fibers in the intrinsic muscle tissue, contractures due to necrosis and fibrosis of the muscle fibers in NMDs, biomechanical analysis of the movement, and normal joint range of the motion and flexibility should be assessed for tracking the disease progression. The range of motion of the joint is monitored objectively by goniometric measurements at regular intervals. The active and passive normal range of the motion should certainly be assessed. The physiotherapist should maintain a record of the presence of limitation and whether the limitation is due to the muscle, the joint capsule, the tendon, or the pain and make a comparison of the agonist-antagonist flexibility. The physiotherapist should consider this situation in the treatment program. In muscle-induced limitations, shortness of muscles should be particularly assessed, particularly since the shortness of hip and knee flexors, plantar flexors, lumbar extensors, latissimus dorsi, pectoral muscles, tensor fascia latae, and quadratus lumborum muscles are considered functional.

Assessment of Motor Function

There are some tests evaluating motor function in NMDs. "Motor Function Measurement (MFM)" is a scale with demonstrated validity and reliability developed to evaluate motor function in all NMDs. It was indicated that this is a scale, which evaluates the severity of motor impairment in the NMD group with good psychometric properties. It was indicated that, other scales, MFM is adapted to the severity of deficits at every level in patients who can or cannot walk and that it evaluates all of the head, trunk, lower, and upper extremities. Some of these tests are specific to the disease, while others focus only on one area of the body. The "Spinal Muscle Atrophy Functional Motor Scale" was prepared for SMA patients, the "Amyotrophic Lateral Sclerosis Functional Classification Scale" and the ALS score for patients with ALS, and the "Hammersmith Motor Skill Score" for patients with DMD. Among the scales focusing only on one region/function of the body, Trunk Control Test and Trunk Impairment Scale are for the trunk, the "Brooke Upper Extremity Scale" is for upper extremity, the "Vignos Lower Extremity Scale" is for lower extremity, the "North Star Ambulatory Assessment" is for ambulation and the "Jebsen-Taylor Hand Function Test" and "Activlim" are for the hand functions.

Performance Tests

The timed and controlled tests of the subsequent tests applied to the patient, evaluating the patient's ability to perform a specific activity in a specific time interval. These include some activities such as rolling from the supine to the prone position, rolling from the prone to the supine position, rising to the sitting position from the lying position, standing up without sitting, walking 10 m, climbing 10 steps up and down, and putting on a t-shirt and taking it off. The Minnesota, Purdue pegboard, nine-hole peg test, and Jebsen hand skill tests were developed and are the most frequently used timed tests to assess hand functions. There are no average values for the timed performance tests. The results are interpreted by comparing the clinical findings with the subsequent tests administered to the patient.

Fatigue

Two different methods are used in fatigue evaluations: electrophysiological tests and scales. Since electrophysiological tests are expensive, scales are more commonly used in clinics. The Multidimensional Fatigue Inventory (MFI), the Fatigue Severity Scale, the Piper Fatigue Scale (PFS), the Short Fatigue Questionnaire (SFQ), the Chalder Fatigue Scale (CSF), Fatigue Impact Scale (FIS), and Visual Analog Scale (VAS) are among the scales used for assessment of fatigue. While each of these tests has its advantages and disadvantages and is used in a large population of patients, none of the tests have been specifically developed for neuromuscular patients.

Respiratory Function

The most commonly used evaluation methods in the clinic are the pulmonary function tests including spirometric measurements of "forced vital capacity (FVC)" and maximum inspiratory and expiratory pressures (MIP, MEP). Cardiopulmonary exercise tests are the evaluation of respiratory muscle strength, thoracic environment measurements, and assessment of respiratory frequency. In the literature, the recommendations on which respiratory evaluation should frequently be done in neuromuscular disease are given in table.

Table: Respiratory follow-up of patients with NMD.

Test	Frequency
History, physical examination	Six monthly and in acute conditions.
Lung function test (FVC, FEV1, VC—upright and supine)	Six monthly and after acute conditions.
MIP, MEP	Six monthly and after acute conditions.
Cough peak expiratory flow	Six monthly and after acute conditions.
Polysomnography	At least yearly, symptom oriented and after acute conditions.

Assessment of Cardiac Functions

Symptoms of heart disease seen in NMDs depend on the severity of skeletal muscle insufficiency and the severity and type of effect. The degree of neuromuscular insufficiency may modulate the symptoms of heart involvement and over time and may sometimes suppress these symptoms. The most commonly used screening test in clinic has two types: resting electrocardiography (ECG) and ambulatory ECG (Holter). Cardiac rhythm, intraventricular state, and ectopic beats can be evaluated noninvasively with

ECG. In particular, cardiopulmonary exercise tests in individuals with severe neuromuscular disease generally show a decrease in maximal oxygen consumption, a decrease in pulmonary ventilation, a reduction in work capacity, and an elevation of resting heart rate. These findings reflect respiratory muscle involvement, cardiac decay, and poor physical fitness.

Pain

The characteristics of the pain should be recorded, such as localization, type, frequency, day-night difference, factors that increase or decrease the pain, change in pain with movement, and the presence of a response to a pain reliever. It should be established which of the causing factors of the pain are involved such as muscle imbalance, trigger points, joint tension, and muscle spasm. One-dimensional and multidimensional scales are used to assess pain severity. One-dimensional scales are intended to measure pain intensity directly, and the patients make the assessment themselves. They are used especially in the evaluation of acute pain and in monitoring the efficacy of applied pain reliever. Among the one-dimensional scales are the verbal category, numerical and visual comparison scale, and Burford Pain Thermometer. Multidimensional scales are thought to be useful in certain cases to assess all aspects of pain in chronic pain. These include the McGill Melzack Pain Questionnaire, the Dartmouth Pain Questionnaire, the West Haven-Yale Multidimensional Pain Inventory, the Memorial Pain Assessment Card, the Wisconsin Brief Pain Inventory, the Pain Perception Profile, and the Behavioral Models.

Assessment of Aerobic (Functional) Capacity

The purpose of evaluating functional capacity is to assess whether or not the maximal or submaximal activities can be performed in nonclinical settings. The ultimate standard to evaluate the person's aerobic exercise response is maximal increasing cardiopulmonary exercise test. A suitable cardiopulmonary exercise test allows determining the underlying pathophysiological mechanisms. These mechanisms include broad assessment of the exercise response, the objective determination of the functional capacity and impairment, the measurement of the appropriate intensity required for long-term exercise, the amount of factors limiting exercise, and the contribution of various organ systems involved in exercise. Functional capacity is assessed by maximal cardiopulmonary exercise tests, motorized treadmill, and stationary bicycle ergometer. However, submaximal tests are recommended in situations where maximal testing increases the patient's risk status and hinders his/her potential abilities, especially in individuals with significant risk for cardiovascular problems, and in cases where multiple cases are to be tested. The 6- or 12-min walking test is a form of submaximal exercise assessment, finds extensive use in the field, is employed in pulmonary diseases and heart disorders, and evaluates the response to various treatment interventions especially pharmacological treatments and exercise training. The ability to walk at a specified distance is a quick, simple, and inexpensive way to evaluate physical function. Walking is also a critical important component of the quality of life because it is highly necessary to accomplish the daily life activities and reflects patient's capacity. The validity study of the 2-min walk test has been conducted in neuromuscular diseases, and it was put to use in recent years since its period of implementation is short and it does not cause fatigue.

Assessment of Functional Mobility and Falling

In clinical practice, the activity and participation problems are also encountered as a result of disorders seen in body structure and function in neuromuscular diseases according to ICF. However, walking emerges as a function related to all of ICF sub-parameters (body structure and functions, activity, participation, personal and environmental factors). In particular, two important conditions must be considered for mobility evaluation according to ICF: the *capacity* is the ability of an individual to perform a function or a task and what the individual is capable of doing in his/her environment is the performance.

Functional mobility, bed mobility, transfer, transfer grounds, gait, and wheelchair should be evaluated. The physiotherapist should assess the level of effort to initiate movement, weight transfer, postural alignment, motion timing and motion completion, patient balance, support surface, walking assistance, and energy expenditure level. The Rivearmed Mobility index is also used in mobility analysis. Walking analysis is done by observational and three-dimensional analysis methods. Some parameters and assessments may be used to analyze the gait. These parameters include step-length asymmetry, position of the ankle during heel strike, knee angle in heel strike, knee flexion angle in stance phase, single extremity support, state of foot and ankle in push phase, knee flexion in swing phase, body position, presence of Trendelenburg sign in frontal plane, knee cap in transverse plane, and foot angle and arm posture. The evaluation should be advanced to investigate possible causes in case of detection of a possible impairment in these standards. For three-dimensional analysis, computerized video cameras, passively reflected signal indicators, multicomponent power platforms, dynamic electromyographic analysis, and temporospatial gait analysis systems are used. The timed-up-and-go test, 30-s chair-stand test, the 4-Stage Balance test, and risk analysis tools such as the Fall Risk Assessment Tool and STRATIFY (St. Thomas Risk Assessment Tool) may be used for the evaluation of falling in neuromuscular diseases. However, there is no specific cutoff value for NMDs in these tests.

Evaluation of Activities of Daily Living (ADL)

Functional level deteriorates due to progressive muscle weakness in NMD, and dependence in ADL increases, while the tests such as Barthel, Katz, and Lawton are used for clinical evaluation of ADL in neurological patients. FIM is the most preferred method for determining the levels of ADL in NMD. The advantage of FIM is that it has proven validity and reliability in evaluating many diseases and that it was found highly reliable by practitioners even when implemented by specialists with varying education and experience.

Sensory Evaluation

In neuromuscular diseases with sensory involvement, especially in peripheral neuropathy, there is a need for frequent sensory evaluation. Surface sensations such as light touch (cotton), pain (sharp-blunt test), and sense of temperature (with hot-cold) and deep sensations such as vibration sensation, pressure recognition, touch localization, joint position, and motion sense should be evaluated.

General Health Measurements

These measurement methods give a general profile of health such as well-being, functions, social, and emotional health. The most commonly used assessments in NMD in this group are "Nottingham Health Profile (NSP)" and the Short Form SF-36 Quality of Life Survey.

Aim and Content of the Rehabilitation Program

Although there have been some promising studies recently, there is no known curative approach to NMD. Physiotherapy and rehabilitation programs are gaining importance to maintain muscle strength, functional capacity, and quality of life as long as possible and to keep the patient in social life. The lack of therapeutic approaches that can curb the progression of the disease in a large proportion of neuromuscular diseases increases the importance of preventive, supportive, compensatory, and rehabilitative approaches. The aim of physiotherapy rehabilitation approaches is to improve the quality of life of patients and their families. Applications in that direction are to delay muscle weakness or loss of strength, to prevent muscle shortness and distortion in joints, to prevent respiratory problems, to maintain the walking activity for as long as possible, to educate the family, to support and keep the function at different stages of the disease, and to increase functional capacity. The rehabilitation program should include the protection of the functional level of the patient and the physical and psychological functions, increasing the physical and mental capacity of the patient, and slowing the progress of the disease symptoms. Patients have a significant number of clinical problems, so rehabilitation should be done with a multidisciplinary team.

The characteristics of the physiotherapist present in the rehabilitation team of neuromuscular patients.

The effectiveness of the rehabilitation program to be administered in NMDs depends on the ability of physiotherapists to assess and analyze the main causes of the patient's problems. As a prominent member of the rehabilitation team, the physiotherapists who will evaluate and implement the rehabilitation in NMD should be specialized for this group of patients and should be able to individualize the rehabilitation program. The physiotherapist should be able to identify the needs of NMD and be able to individualize the treatment program based on needs. The physiotherapist should have knowledge about the pathophysiology of the disorders in the patient and about the progression of the disease. The physiotherapist should be able to serve in different settings (inpatient and outpatient clinics, at home, at home-care facilities, and in workplace arrangements) and various age groups. The physiotherapist should be able to follow up the patient with the short/long-span controls during the planning of research on NMD, the development and implementation of outcome measurements, the setting of treatment interventions, and the natural progression of the disease and should be able to document the process well.

The rehabilitation program should include the muscle strength preservation, an exercise program for the prevention of contractures, increasing in respiratory function, increasing the functional (aerobic) capacity, walking and balance training, fall prevention and the stages of deciding walking aids, nutrition expert support, psychosocial approach, vocational counseling, and ergotherapy processes.

Preservation of Muscle Strength and Prevention of Contractures

Many international researchers agree on the use of exercise therapy in neuromuscular diseases. There are many physical and psychological benefits of exercise such as muscle strength preservation, prevention of contractures, increased flexibility, reduced energy expenditure, relieving fatigue, reducing pain, depression, social isolation and loneliness, ensuring the participation of the individual active life, sustaining mobility, and increasing the quality of life. However, the number of studies with a high level of evidence about type, intensity, frequency, and speed of the exercise is limited. When deciding on a possible exercise program, the pathophysiology, onset, severity and the progression of the disease, the age and sex of the patient, and the intensity and frequency of the exercise to be given should be considered. In general, there is a consensus on the positive effects of mild to moderate exercise programs on muscular strength without causing significant muscle damage, particularly in the early stages of neuromuscular disease with moderate progress when the muscle strength was not severely affected. Combined use of upper/lower extremity exercises with neck and body exercises is preferred in clinical practice due to the ability to spread force from strong muscles to weak muscles and relieve fatigue.

Stretching and Normal Range-of-Motion Exercises

Stretching and normal range-of-motion exercises can prevent the limitation of joint mobility that develops as secondary to the muscle weakness. The static stretching, which is usually used for treatment in NMDs, is performed by proper alignment of the joint and bringing the muscle to its maximum length along the joint during stabilization of the unmovement joints. When the movement reaches the end, the position is held for at least 10 s and repeated. Although healthy individuals are recommended to make one to two repetitions a day or three to seven repetitions per week regarding the frequency of stretching, there is no definite information for neuromuscular patients. Daily stretching exercises are recommended. It has been reported that ROM increases with stretching frequency and the improvement was maintained for 4 weeks after the exercise ends. Surveys show that a little 5-min static stretching causes a change in the muscle-tendon unit. Resting splints can be used during sleep to prevent contractures. When bed confinement has developed, lower extremities can be stretched using the body weight with standing table.

Strength Training

Strength training can be done with resistance exercises. Resistance exercise training is one of the most effective ways to improve the functional capacity of the neuromuscular system. However, the potential benefits and risks of strength training in neuromuscular diseases are still a controversial subject in the literature. Progressive strengthening exercises are also commonly used to increase muscle strength in neuromuscular diseases. Progressive strengthening exercises improve lean body mass, muscle protein mass, contractile strength, strength, and physical function. This improvement varies according to the rate of progression of the disease. There is a consensus in recent years about the benefits of mild to moderate intensity strength training (25–40% of maximum weight) on muscle strength without any deleterious effects, especially for slow-progressing neuromuscular diseases. Considering that the high-intensity (50–70% of maximum weight) eccentric -or concentric- type exercise programs would cause mechanical stress on muscle fibers and increase muscle weakness, they are not recommended for use on dystrophic types with rapid progression and membrane instability (such as Duchenne muscular dystrophy). However, studies with opposite point of view also exist suggesting that high-intensity training is beneficial with appropriate selection of patients. However, no additional contribution to muscle strength and endurance was shown in a comparison of the maximum intensity weight training to the medium- and low-intensity weight training.

Strengthening principles applied especially in healthy muscles should be used carefully here. The level of intensity and resistance, which is above the patient's muscle strength, strain the patient, and cause muscle fatigue, should be avoided. The patient should be recommended to do the exercises in parts during the day so as not to cause fatigue. It should be started with little or no resistance and few repetitions, and the frequency, duration, and resistance of the exercise should be monitored with monthly or tri-monthly evaluations. The intensity and resistance of exercise should be revised if the patient experiences pain, muscle spasms, fasciculations, and excessive fatigue after exercises.

Electrical stimulation commonly used in the clinic for strengthening should also be used with caution in NMDs. Since all muscle fibers contract at the same time with electrical stimulation, it can increase degeneration in patients with low muscle fiber counts.

For this reason, patients with muscle strength below three should use current types that will not cause fatigue.

In-water Exercises (Aqua Therapy)

In-water exercises are the most appropriate exercise method for this group of patients. The water lift supports weakened muscles, permits functional movement, and in some cases can also be used as a resistance exercise. Pool exercises treat all muscle groups and maximize the aerobic capacity of the patient. It is particularly effective in a group of patients with limited energy levels. It is recommended in the literature to apply 45 min twice a week. Limitations of pool therapy are lack of accessibility and insurance payment.

Aerobic Endurance Training

Aerobic endurance training generates physiological responses that are different from strength training. Sufficient intensity and duration for aerobic training that involves the use of large muscle groups and will not cause fatigue is 50–85% of VO2max and 30 min. Aerobic training causes stimulation in the heart, the peripheral circulation, and the musculoskeletal system. As a result, circulation of more oxygen in the body leads to an increase in cardiac output, capillary density, and vascular transmission. For this benefit, aerobic exercises such as swimming, walking, and cycling can be performed, which put fewer burdens on the musculoskeletal system.

According to the American College of Sports Medicine guidelines, it is adequate to improve cardiorespiratory fitness for most aerobic training when an optimal frequency of 70–85% of maximum heart rate and 60–80% of maximum oxygen consumption are combined with an optimal frequency of 3–5 days per week. An aerobic training at this intensity can be recommended to the NMD patients with a good functional level. In most of the studies included in the review, the cycling or treadmill exercises done at least three times a week and the use of approximately 70% of the heart rate reserve or the use of an estimated maximum heart rate are recommended. It is stated that the whole program lasting at least 10 weeks for both muscle strengthening and aerobic exercises and regular physical therapist supervision increases the effectiveness and improves the safety and suitability of the exercise. However, in only 30% of all studies involving muscle strengthening and aerobic exercises, training lasted for less than 10 weeks, with an average of 5 weeks. In the literature, it is indicated that the aerobic exercise training in conjunction with muscle strengthening exercises is effective at evidence level of 2 or 3, especially in muscle diseases and neuromuscular patients with heterogeneous features.

Development of Postural Control

The activity of coming to sitting position from the supine position is an important activity of the body against the gravity and is one of the first stages of mobility. During this activity, which is very important for muscle patients also, the anterior trunk muscles contract concentrically while the posterior trunk muscles contract eccentrically. The difficulty of the patient in coming to the sitting position should bring into mind the possibility of encountering mobility problems and that the treatment should involve the precautions related to the trunk.

The equilibrium reactions have been tested in patients with isolated muscle weakness, and it was concluded that the muscle weakness is important. Although patients with distal leg weakness are particularly prone to stumble-like stability disorders, the stability has been observed to decrease following the external perturbations of balance in proximal muscle weakness. In previous studies, it has been shown that balance correction strategies assessed by dynamic posturography can vary depending on body parts where muscle weakness is present. Some muscle responses are sensitive to balance perturbations, especially in the sagittal (anterior-posterior) plane, while others are found to be sensitive to the frontal plane or a combination of these two planes. This reveals that the proximal and axial muscles (such as paraspinal or gluteus medius) are more frontal-focused, the lower-limb muscles are more sagittal-focused sensitivity, and the knee muscles have the sensitive role in both directions in muscle response sensitivities following proximal to distal disturbances. Therefore, the patient maintains the balance based on these sided sensitivities, and the question whether the patients with distal muscle weakness are more distressed in the sagittal plane and those with proximal lower extremity weakness are more distressed in the frontal plane should be answered. It is thought that this information can also help in the planning of therapeutic interventions. For example, patients with complete proximal weakness are unstable in balance correction strategies associated with the frontal plane; these patients will need a different intervention than those with complete distal weakness and possibly unstable in strategies associated with the sagittal plane.

Increasing Respiratory Capacity

If there is a coughing weakness in the patient, airway cleaning techniques such as air stacking (glossopharyngeal breathing), mechanical, and manual coughing should be applied as soon as possible. Increasing the pulmonary capacity, breathing exercises, diaphragm breathing exercises, and thoracic expansion exercises aim to maximize the expansion of the patients' lungs and should be taught to the patient.

Pulmonary expansion therapy and maximal insufflation therapy (mask or mechanically assisted hyperinsufflation) increase the forced inspiratory vital capacity. It is reported in the literature that maximum insufflation therapy is important in increasing peak cough flow for neuromuscular patients with vital capacities less than 1500 mL. Manually supported coughing techniques should be continued for maximum expansion. Secretion mobilization can also be provided by a positive expiratory pressure device. With a positive expiratory pressure device, patients breathe freely and breathe against a moderate resistance; air pressure activates secretions, preventing atelectasis.

Traditional chest physiotherapy techniques used for airway cleaning should be taught to this patient population. This involves taking the patient to different positions, then clapping on the chest wall, vibrating, and coughing. However, it should be taken into account that Trendelenburg, lateral recumbent, and prone positions are difficult to tolerate in NMDs.

Mechanical Insufflation-Exsufflation (Assisted Coughing Device)

The assisted coughing device operates according to the principle of vacuum cleaning. Cleansing of strong expiratory flow and secretions is achieved without tracheostomy by applying negative pressure after maximal insufflation with a positive pressure of the oronasal mask. It is also known to be more effective than aspiration catheters in tracheostomized patients. The use of a peak cough flow below 160 L/min in NMDs is found appropriate. However, a cough flow of at least 300 L/min was used to initiate maximum assisted mechanical cough assistance. The assisted coughing device produces an airflow of approximately 10 L/s with pressures between -40 cm HO_2 and 40 cm HO_2. It is a very vital and efficient device to use in patients using a mechanical ventilator and has reduced coughing ability. Noninvasive mechanical ventilation devices are employed in later stages of NMDs.

Reduction of Pain

The mechanism of pain has not been identified in detail in neuromuscular patients. For this reason, the physiotherapist should choose the appropriate treatment modality based on the pain source he/she has identified. From among the physiotherapy techniques, ultrasound, TENS, hot/cold application, and massage may be used but there are very few studies on the effectiveness of these techniques. There are even contradictory results regarding the increased muscle destruction of the ultrasound and hot application. Physiotherapists should be so cautious in their use. It is thought that TENS is preferred because it uses different ways of inhibiting pain.

In the loss of muscle strength, joint pain can often be associated with improper alignment or excessive stretching of the joint capsule. Pain relief is possible with proper alignment of the joint and removal of excessive tension. However, since the weakness of each NMD patient is seen in different forms, it should be analyzed well before choosing the appropriate treatment. External support such as splints can be used when muscle weakness makes self-stabilization impossible. An external shoulder splint may be utilized for the shoulder pain resulting from shoulder subluxation while an abdominal mattress may be preferred for back pain due to the excessive weakening of the abdominal muscles.

Shoulder pain may arise due to the single-point cane, which NMD patients often prefer for cosmetic reasons. In this case, a four-point walker may be used if the patient's energy expenditure level is not increased. If the size of the four-point walker is not suitable for the patient and the patient bends forward, this may be a possible reason for back pain. If the patient has a lack of postural control and the arms carry the whole load when the walker is used, this may be considered as a possible cause of pain in the upper extremity. If the patient's upper extremity strength is unable to carry the weight of the walker and the patient has upper extremity and back pain, then the arm-assisted wheeled walker can be used to reduce pain.

The shoulder pain that occurs in patients using wheelchairs may be due to the improperly positioned inadequate arm support, which prevents the alignment of the humerus in the glenohumeral joint, while the hip and back pain may be caused by improper knee-hip level and foot support. Wheelchair cushions, unsuitable pillows, and the bed should be considered as possible reasons for pain. The preference of a pressure distributing bed is also an important factor in reducing pain in bed dependence.

Walking and Balance Training

Mobility target should be determined according to the evaluation and the progression of the disease. Walking training should include endurance training, teaching the use of walking aids, orthotic approach and fall prevention, learning safe-fall techniques, teaching how to stand up after falling, and teaching energy conservation techniques. In NMDs, the level of energy expenditure during walking increases. For this reason, physiotherapists should choose the most appropriate aerobic exercise for the patient; the disease and exercise tolerance should be closely monitored. Physiotherapists should evaluate and recommend ambulatory assistive devices, transfer supports, and orthoses for improved walking, energy conservation, and safety if the patient develops weakness. However, the use of wrong assistive devices may alter the patient's optimal gait pattern and may prevent gait function or cause new problems in the patient. It has been shown that walking aids affect stability in a negative way in a group of studies in the literature.

The reason for stability to be affected is that the upper- and lower-extremity balance reactions, normally used to protect against falls and protective, are restricted by the walking aid. There is also the problem of lower-extremity tripping over the mobility aid. It is stated that the reciprocal movements necessary to use the walking aid in these situations are difficult to achieve. Choosing the right walking aid, using the right size, and training with the walking aid can reduce the risk of falling. Walking aids prevent falls when used safely; it should be kept in mind that they may be the most important reason for falling if misused. When the falling story is evaluated, the frequency of falls, during which activity the fall occurred, the balance, sense, proprioception, the characteristics of the fall area, and the home environment should be evaluated. Balance and proprioception training should be given as a result of these evaluations. Recommendations for orthosis can be made by a physiotherapist, an orthotist, or a doctor. When orthosis advice is given, the desired function, weight, and device tolerance should be considered, and a lightweight material should be used.

The articulated orthoses may be granted if the patient has muscular strength to control the dynamic orthosis, fixed orthoses may be given if not. Walking training should be provided with the orthosis given.

Training for the Activities of Daily Living and Adaptive Approach

It has been shown that there is a negative correlation between manual muscle test results and FIM results in studies performed. The manual muscle test score of 3 is a critical threshold value. The average muscle strength value being 3 is an important indicator that the patient is dependent/independent in the activities of daily living or a candidate for dependence. Weakness in the upper extremities causes patients to lose their independence in basic activities of daily living such as dressing, nutrition, and personal hygiene. In addition, muscle weakness around the shoulder in diseases with more pronounced proximal muscle weakness causes difficulty in performing activities such as shaving, makeup, and weight lifting; distal muscle weakness causes difficulty in gripping and increases the functional deficiencies of patients in activities such as writing, turning the faucet on/off, and unlocking the door with the key. It has been found that the activities indicated by the patients as the most challenging are climbing stairs (72%), taking along walk (40%), and getting on or off the bus (18%).

To be able to perform the activities of daily living independently, the functional capacity of the individual and the environmental conditions necessary to carry out the activity should be able to match fully with each other. When there is a discrepancy between these two parameters, problems arise which affect the quality of life of the person negatively. These problems can be solved by increasing the functional capacity of the individual, reducing environmental demands, and adapting the environment to the individual. For example, if a person needs to pick up any item at the top shelf, he/she should be able to lift his/her arms over his/her shoulder. If he/she cannot lift his/her arms, he/she cannot be considered completely independent of this activity. This problem can be solved by strengthening the shoulder muscles to allow the arms to be raised above the head, or by lowering the height of the shelf with a manually adjustable cabinet to the level at which the patient can lift his/her arms.

Neuromuscular patients need different aids at various periods of the disease to be able to perform their daily life activities independently as the disease progresses. Assistive devices include tools designed or modified to increase the functional capacities of persons with disabilities that can be considered in a broad spectrum. This equipment can range from simple tools such as jar openers, pen holders, electronic environmental control systems, toilet lifts to prevent fatigue, handlebars, forks, and spoons with thickened stalk, and adjustable beds to complex technological tools. Parallel to the developments in technology, assistive devices are also renewed every day. As the complexity and technology increase, the costs of the assistive devices also increase, making it difficult for patients to obtain these devices. Appropriate devices prescribed to a neuromuscular patient increase the patient's quality of life.

Myotonic Dystrophy

Myotonic dystrophy is the most common form of muscular dystrophy in adults. It is an autosomal dominant disorder, which means that a person carrying the gene has a 50-50 chance of passing it on to a child. It is a multi-systemic progressive disorder that affects the muscular, respiratory, cardiac, nervous and endocrine systems. Currently 2 variants of DM are recognized – DM1 which arises from a defect on chromosome 19 and DM2 which results from a defect on chromosome DM1 was first described in the early 1900's and hence is a much better studied entity while DM2 was only described in the past decade and hence there is a lot to learn regarding this phenotype. DM1 and DM2 share many common features, but there are also significant differences. Individuals with DM1 can present with symptoms at different ages; at birth (congenital), during childhood (pediatric), during adulthood, or later in life and thus four clinical phenotypes are described in the literature. Congenital phenotypes have not been described in DM2 yet and most patients present in adulthood. Weakness and wasting (atrophy) are prominent features in DM1 whereas muscle pain and myotonia are prominent in DM2. Individuals with DM1 primarily exhibit facial and distal limb weakness whereas individuals with DM2 exhibit proximal weakness. Muscle related problems - weakness, wasting and functional problems - are very often the concerns that lead individuals to seek attention and help from physical therapists. However, DM is a multi-systemic disorder and hence it is essential to understand all the systemic complaints and help manage the muscle related symptoms in the overall context of concerns for an individual. Congenital and childhood onset DM1 have unique features.

Physical Therapy Assessment

During an initial evaluation a physical therapist will obtain a detailed history of the symptoms and/or problems, how they have changed over time, factors that make them better or worse and how they affect the daily activities and lives of the affected individual. Information regarding the person's occupation, lifestyle, leisure activities, and their role in the family unit is essential to the evaluation process.

Myotonic dystrophy is a systemic condition. It is therefore important for the physical therapist to perform a systems review according to the Guide to Physical Therapy 5 including review of cognition/communication, musculoskeletal system, neuromuscular system, cardiovascular/pulmonary system, and integumentary/skin system.

Individuals with DM can have difficulties in both, cognition and communication. Symptoms include, somnolence, apathy, specific personality traits, deficit in executive functions, depression and fatigue. These cognitive deficits may impact a person's ability to comply with recommendations and are important to take into consideration when establishing a plan of care or management program. Communication difficulties can arise as a result of weakness of the facial muscles as well as the presence of myotonia in the jaw and tongue. This not only impacts proper communication between patients and care providers, but also has an effect on social communication leading to some of the psychosocial issues mentioned previously.

The neuromuscular and musculoskeletal systems are often the focus of the examination, as weakness and resulting functional difficulties are often the most disabling features of the disorder. The most common pattern of muscle involvement in DM1 includes the facial (masseter and temporalis) muscles, neck muscles (sternocleidomastoids), long-finger flexors of the hand and ankle dorsiflexors and/or plantarexors4. Muscle involvement usually begins in the teens, twenties or thirties and is slowly progressive. The weakness progresses from the distal to proximal muscles. Muscular weakness in congenital myotonic dystrophy presents during the neonatal period with generalized hypotonia. In DM2 the muscular involvement is predominantly proximal and also slowly progressive, beginning in the 'mid-adult' life. It is critical that physical therapists are knowledgeable in manual muscle testing for all muscles, as the pattern of weakness can be predictive of both the disease itself as well as mobility concerns that may arise. Strength can also be measured more objectively by hand-held dynamometers as well as expensive systems such as a Quantitative Muscle Assessment (QMA) system. QMA systems are often utilized in the research setting. Normative data for both of these methods have been established in the pediatric as well as adult populations.

Myotonia is the other musculoskeletal manifestation of myotonic dystrophy. Myotonia is the inability to relax a muscle after a forceful contraction. Individuals with myotonia affecting the hand musculature often report difficulty releasing their grip after a vigorous handshake which creates an embarrassing social situation. Complaints of myotonia are also reported in the jaw and tongue leading to difficulties with speech, swallowing and chewing. Myotonia in the leg muscles may lead to difficulty with movements like climbing stairs, running etc. Symptoms of myotonia may also be present in other parts of the body. Often patients will report that their myotonia symptoms are worse in cooler temperatures. Myotonia has been managed with medications such as Mexilitene.

DM1 is a slowly progressive disease and as strength decreases, individuals may become adept in substituting less affected muscles to perform movement. Hence it is important to assess simple functional activities, including the ability to get up from a chair, ambulate and climb stairs. These functional tasks can also be timed and used as outcome measures to document benefits of interventions or to monitor the progression of the disease. Assessment of hand function, including grip and pinch strength, is also important in this population.

The cardiovascular system can be compromised by the presence of cardiac arrhythmias and conduction defects as well as involvement of the cardiac muscle itself. Insufficiency of the respiratory system may be a result of both myotonia and weakness in the muscles that control respiration. Respiratory muscle involvement often leads to a reduced vital capacity later in the disease. Individuals with DM1 who have reduced respiratory function are often at more risk for pulmonary complications such as pneumonia. When making exercise recommendations for a home program, it is essential to educate individuals about how to monitor their cardio respiratory responses with simple tools like pulse monitors, Borg scale, etc. It is essential that individuals report their responses to exercise to the person overseeing and/or monitoring the home program. Depending on the progression of their disease, individuals with myotonic dystrophy may have limited exercise tolerance and will need to be monitored carefully.

The integumentary system is not usually involved as the sensory system is spared in myotonic dystrophy. However, if poor mobility is demonstrated and bony prominences are exposed secondary to muscle wasting, the integumentary system may require attention.

Pain and Fatigue are common complaints among individuals with DM1 and DM2. In a study by Jensen, complaints of pain were reported most commonly in the low back and legs. More than 60% of patients with neuromuscular disorders complain of fatigue. Fatigue can have a major impact on the employment status of patients with DM. Therefore, pain and fatigue should be assessed and addressed in the treatment plan as necessary.

Lastly, it should also be mentioned that many of these individuals have gastrointestinal manifestations that may be present anywhere along the digestive tract. Symptoms reported span the spectrum of dysphasia and heartburn to abdominal pain and changes in bowel function. Involvement of the GI system may be very disabling to the individual and again, may impact the person's ability to participate in exercise programs.

Physical Therapy Management

Exercise

Individuals with myotonic dystrophy often have questions about exercise. Exercise, including range of motion, strengthening and cardiovascular (aerobic) exercise, is important for the management of the musculoskeletal and cardiorespiratory manifestations of myotonic dystrophy. Range of motion exercises are important in maintaining joint function and muscular balance and may play a role in reducing pain that is caused by muscular imbalance or tightness. As muscles atrophy resulting in weakness, gravitational pull may limit a person's ability to move a body part through its entire range of motion and therefore it may be important to change the position of the body part to minimize the pull of gravity. For example, people may have difficulty raising their arms up in sitting or standing position, i.e. performing shoulder abduction in an antigravity position, but may have the ability to perform this movement when lying down in a supine position where gravity is eliminated. Individuals may also participate in range of motion exercises that are more dynamic in nature. This includes Yoga and Pilates based activities that can either be done individually or in a class setting. Education regarding range of motion exercise is essential to the management of the symptoms related to the musculoskeletal system.

Weakness occurs as part of the disease process; however, weakness may also develop secondary to disuse. Strengthening exercises may help to minimize the disuse weakness; but there is also a concern that too much exercise or inappropriate exercise may hasten disease progression, and hence finding the right balance for each individual is important. The evidence available regarding the role of exercise in myotonic dystrophy is limited. In a Cochrane study published in 2010. The authors examined the safety and efficacy of strength and aerobic training in neuromuscular diseases. They identified a total of 36 studies; however, there were only three randomized controlled trials that fulfilled their inclusion criteria. Based on these studies the authors concluded that strengthening exercises at a moderate intensity did not worsen the disease progression in persons with myotonic dystrophy. Many of the studies involving individuals with myotonic dystrophy were excluded from the study because they lacked randomization. Many of these studies also grouped different neuromuscular diseases together, making it difficult to draw conclusions about the individual's response to exercise in a specific disease like DM. Disorders like DM are difficult to study as they are rare diseases and it is difficult to enrol enough patients to carry out a well powered randomized control trial. Other problems cited with the reviewed studies included lack of detailed descriptions of the exact exercise protocols used and short durations of the exercise trials. Or green and colleagues studied the benefits of aerobic exercise using bicycle ergo meters in patients with DM1 and concluded that aerobic exercise is safe and improves fitness in patients with DM1. Cup. chose to look at the evidence related to exercise in individuals with neuromuscular diseases with expanded criteria than those in the Cochrane reviews. Based on their analysis of the studies they concluded that the evidence suggests that strengthening exercises in combination with aerobic exercises are "likely to be effective". Given the evidence from the 2 major reviews that exercise may be effective and that moderate exercise does not worsen disease progression, some general recommendations regarding exercise can be made to guide clinicians and individuals with myotonic dystrophy.

Depending on the activity level of the individuals, they may benefit from a strengthening program. Individuals who lead an active lifestyle may not have much disuse weakness, and further activity may be fatiguing to them. However, others who lead a more sedentary lifestyle may benefit from a strengthening program. Strengthening exercise can be accomplished in several ways with resistance provided by gravity, water – in a pool - or equipment such as elastic bands, free weights and machines. Yoga and Pilates types of exercises may also be recommended as part of a strengthening program, but there are no studies reported that have examined the effects of these specific interventions in patients with DM. It is essential that individuals with myotonic dystrophy work with providers knowledgeable about their condition; have proper baseline evaluation and appropriate follow-up to monitor and modify the program as necessary.

Cardiovascular exercise performed at a low to moderate intensity has been found to be safe in people with myotonic dystrophy. Cup et al. also concluded that there was "indication of effectiveness" for aerobic exercises in individuals with muscle disorders. However, because of the cardiac involvement that can occur in persons with myotonic dystrophy, it is essential that individuals have a physical, appropriate cardiac evaluations and clearance from their primary care physicians prior to initiating an aerobic exercise program.

Current recommendations from the U.S Department of Health and Human Services (HHS) suggest that for all individuals, some activity is better than none and that the health benefits of physical activity far outweigh the risks. They recommend that children, adolescents, adults (ages 18-64) and older adults follow the appropriate guidelines to the best of their ability. Individuals with chronic conditions perform as much activity and/or exercise as their condition allows. These include about 2 hours and 30 minutes a week of moderate intensity exercise. Aerobic exercise should be performed in episodes of at least 10 minutes preferably spread throughout the week. Muscle strengthening activities that involve all major muscle groups should be performed at least 2-3 days a week.

Examples of moderate intensity activities include – walking briskly, biking on level ground or on a stationary bicycle, ballroom and line dancing, general gardening, household activities, canoeing, using hand cycles, using a manual wheelchair and water aerobics. Moderate exercises are activities that you can perform while still continuing a conversation –without having to stop to catch your breath.

Pain

A wide variety of methods have been used in the treatment of pain in individuals with myotonic dystrophy. The use of non-steroidal anti-inflammatory medications or acetaminophen, exercise (strengthening and ROM), and heat are the most common therapies used to manage pain. Individuals should consult their physician for recommendations regarding the use of medication for pain relief.

Fatigue

Currently there are no reports of specific interventions and their impact on management of fatigue in patients with DM. Interventions may need to be individualized based on specific factors contributing to the complaint of fatigue.

Orthotics

Lower extremity weakness can affect a person's ability to walk safely, especially on uneven surfaces. Ankle dorsiflexion weakness often leads to a foot drop and decreased foot clearance during the swing phase of gait. Some individuals may compensate for the ankle dorsiflexion weakness by using a steppage gait pattern, i.e. lifting their knees higher to help the foot clear the ground. The use of ankle-foot-orthotics can help to correct the foot drop; however, care must be taken in prescribing an AFO. Several factors may play a role in the effectiveness of orthotic use in the lower extremities. The additional weight that may be added to the lower extremity by a brace can significantly alter the person's ability to ambulate, and hence it is important that the orthotics are made of the lightest materials available. It is also important to consider the person's ability to don and doff the orthotic devices, especially in the presence of hand weakness and decreased hand function. Orthotic fit is often difficult because people with myotonic dystrophy have muscular wasting, and bony landmarks often become more prominent and susceptible to skin irritation and breakdown. Comfort and satisfaction are important in promoting the use of the prescribed device. Compliance suffers if the prescribed orthotic device is uncomfortable or too difficult for the client to get on and off independently. Furthermore, there has been very limited research on the effect of orthotic use on energy expenditure during walking and is definitely an area that needs further investigation to prescribe appropriate orthotics to this patient population. In cases where the neck muscles are also affected, neck braces may also be beneficial. Many of these braces are off the shelf and can be fit by an orthotist.

Assistive Devices/Adaptive Equipment

Individuals with myotonic dystrophy are at a higher risk for falls. Decreased visual acuity, lower extremity weakness and depression can play a role in increasing the risk for stumbles and falls. The use of canes, walkers, wheelchairs, and powered mobility devices can be used to allow a person to continue to be safe and independent in mobility. Adaptive equipment, such as long handled sponges, foam buildups on silverware and pens, and button hooks can make performing bathing and dressing easier and allow individuals to be more independent in caring for themselves. When assessing for adaptive equipment, a referral to an occupational therapist may also be beneficial.

Children with Myotonic Dystrophy

Even though DM1 is considered the most common of the adult muscular dystrophies, congenital (present at birth) and childhood presentations are recognized. Congenital myotonic dystrophy tends to be more severe than the childhood form and is often associated with hypotonia, respiratory insufficiency and feeding problems. When symptoms arise during the childhood years, the progression is similar to that in adult onset myotonic dystrophy, however since the symptoms start earlier, they may be more severe later in life. Cognitive impairment is also present in these phenotypes, with the involvement being more severe in the congenital form. The need for physical therapy services can be highly variable and individualized based on the type and severity of the symptoms. The areas addressed by physical therapists will be the same as in the adult population, including recommendations regarding exercise, orthotics, and adaptive equipment. Additionally, the child will be developing motor skills, and there may be a need for short episodes of intensive hands on therapy to facilitate motor development and attainment of motor milestones. Hands on physical therapy services can be provided in several different settings including home, daycare, school, playground and clinic depending on the goals of the therapy session. In addition to typical interventions such as range of motion and strengthening exercises, practice of activities of daily living, motor skill development, therapy may include aquatic therapy or hippotherapy - the utilization of equine movement.

Aquatic therapy uses the physical properties of water to perform exercise. The buoyancy provides support and facilitates movements. The viscosity or resistive properties of the water allow for strengthening of the postural and limb muscles. These qualities of the aquatic environment have been shown to be benecial in improving functional mobility of children with mobility limitations. Hippotherapy is another treatment strategy in which the movement of a horse is used to address impairments and functional limitations in people with neuromuscular dysfunction. Hippotherapy has been shown to improve upright posture, and balance therefore positively impacting gross motor function and walking ability in children with developmental delay.

There are no reports of any studies that have looked specically at using aquatherapy or hippotherapy in children with myotonic dystrophy. It is dicult to document the specic impact of these interventions versus the natural gains that occur with development since there are very few appropriately controlled longitudinal case studies reported in the literature. Hence further research is needed to determine the appropriate type, frequency, intensity, and duration of physical therapy services in children with myotonic dystrophy.

Currently, the frequency and intensity of the hands on services vary depending on the individual child's needs. These may be followed by more limited episodes where the physical therapist will play a more consultative role, monitoring the child's development and working with the family to set up a home based program of daily activities and exercises to maximize the child's functional abilities. Within the school system, the physical therapist will work with the school team – classroom teachers, gym teachers, school nurse, and counselors etc educating them regarding the condition and the appropriate activities and supports within the school environment to assure safety, mobility and maximize the learning opportunities.

References

- Neuromuscular-disorders, health-conditionsandtreatments: betterhealth.vic.gov.au, Retrieved 17 January, 2019

- Types-of-neuromuscular-disorders, discover-md: muscle.ca, Retrieved 09 June, 2019

- Neuromuscular-diseases-and-rehabilitation, neurological-physical-therapy: intechopen.com, Retrieved 25 August, 2019

- Myofascial-pain: now.aapmr.org, Retrieved 23 July, 2019

- Strength training and aerobic exercise training for muscle disease. The Cochrane Library. 2010; 2

Chapter 4

Pediatric Rehabilitation Medicine

The field of medicine which aims to prevent, detect, treat and manage congenital and childhood-onset physical disabilities is referred to as pediatric rehabilitation medicine. It includes pediatric muscular dystrophies, pediatric neurorehabilitation medicine, rehabilitation management, etc. All these diverse aspects of pediatric rehabilitation medicine have been carefully analyzed in this chapter.

Pediatric Neuromuscular Disorders

The neuromuscular system includes all muscles throughout the body and the nerves that connect them. There are a wide variety of neuromuscular disorders that can occur in children. These conditions impact the peripheral nervous system, which includes the muscles, neuromuscular (nerve-muscle) junction, peripheral nerves in the limbs and motor-nerve cells in the spinal cord.

There are many types of neuromuscular disorders, including:

Brachial Plexopathy

This is a condition in which there is damage on each side of the neck where the nerve roots from the spinal cord split into the nerves for each arm.

Charcot-Marie-Tooth Syndrome

CMT is an inherited neurological disorder that often causes problems with walking, speaking, breathing and swallowing.

Chronic Inflammatory Demyelinating Polyneuropathy

CIDP is a neurological disorder that causes progressive weakness and reduced function in the arms and legs.

Congenital Myopathy

Congenital myopathies are a group of rare, congenital (present at birth) muscle diseases that are caused by genetic defects.

Guillain-Barre Syndrome

Guillain-Barre syndrome causes the body's immune system to attack the nerves, which can eventually lead to paralysis throughout the body.

Muscular Dystrophy

Muscular dystrophy is an inherited, genetic condition that causes weakness in the muscle and usually shows signs in the first few years of a child's life.

Myasthenia Gravis

Myasthenia gravis causes weakness and rapid fatigue of the muscles over which a person normally has control.

Cerebral Palsy

Pediatric Rehabilitation requires a Multi-disciplianary (MDT) Approach in order to promote the independence of the child with an impairment, both functionally and psychologically and increase the quality of life of both the child and their family. Physiotherapists, viewed as the 'movement expert', play a key role within this MDT. The main aim of Physiotherapy, is to support the child with Cerebral Palsy to achieve their potential for physical independence and fitness levels within their community, by minimising the effect of their physical impairments, and to improve the quality of life of the child and their family who have major role to play in the process.

Physiotherapy focuses on function, movement, and optimal use of the child's potential and uses physical approaches to promote, maintain and restore physical, psychological and social well-being within all environments of the child including home, school, recreation, and community environments.

Gross motor skills, functional mobility in the management for the motor deficits, positioning, sitting, transition from sitting to standing, walking with or without assistive devices and orthoses, wheelchair use and transfers, are all areas that the physiotherapist works on using a wide range of physiotherapeutic approaches to influence functional ability of the child.

Treatment Approaches

A wide range of therapeutic interventions have been used in the treatment and management of children with cerebral palsy. They show that there is evidence to support the use and effectiveness of neuromuscular electrical stimulation, while evidence in support of the effectiveness of the neurodevelopmental treatment is equivocal at best. The effectiveness of many other interventions, including include: sensory integration, body-weight support treadmill training, conductive education, constraint-induced therapy, hyperbaric oxygen therapy used in the treatment of cerebral palsy have not been clearly established based on well-controlled trials.

A wide range of choices and availability of various techniques which may vary both between therapists and from country to country.

Therapeutic approach to the management of CP:

- Bobath/Neurodevelopmental therapy (NDT),
- Conductive education,
- Sensory integration,
- Adeli suit,
- Aim-oriented management,
- Advance neuromotor rehabilitation,
- Biofeedback,
- Dohsa-Hou (a Japanese psychorehabilitation technique),
- Electrical stimulation,
- Early intervention (e. g. Portage project),
- Functional physical therapy,
- Movement Opportunities via Education (MOVE),
- Patterning (Doman-Delacato, i.e.IAHP/BIBIC/Brainwave),
- Pelvic positioning,
- Physical activity training,
- Strength training Targeted training,
- Vojta,
- Training program (15 modalities) by Phelps,
- Recreational therapies (e.g. hippotherapy /saddle riding, hydrotherapy/swimming programmes),
- Alternative therapies (e.g. hyperbaric oxygen therapy, acupuncture, and osteocraniosacral therapy).

Neurodevelopmental Treatment

One of the more popular approaches utilised in the management of cerebral palsy, the NDT Approach also know as Bobath Approach, was developed in the 1940's by Berta and Karl Bobath, based on their personal observations working with children with cerebral palsy. The basis of this approach is that motor abnormalities seen in children with Cerebral Palsy are due to atypical development in relation to postural control and reflexes because of the underlying dysfunction of the central nervous system. This approach aims to facilitate typical motor development and function and to prevent development of secondary impairments due to muscle contractures, joint and limb deformities. Although the effectiveness of NDT in Cerebral Palsy has been questioned by some published reports, there are some studies suggesting its effectiveness.

Constraint-induced Movement Therapy

Constraint-induced Movement therapy is used predominantly in the individual with Hemiplegic Cerebral Palsy to improve the use of the affected upper limb. The stronger or non-impaired upper limb is immobilized for a variable duration in order to Force Use of the impaired upper limb over time. Antilla et al (2008) identified one high and one lower-quality trials which measured both body functions and structures, and activity and participation outcomes through use of CIMT. Use of a cast with CIMT showed positive effects in the amount and quality of functional hand use in the impaired limb and new emerging behaviour as compared to the no-therapy group, but no effects were found on QUEST. Use of sling during CIMT also had positive effects on functional hand use on the impaired upper limb, time to complete tasks, and speed and dexterity, but no effects on sensibility, handgrip force, or spasticity. Thus Antilla et al (2005) found there is moderate evidence for the effectiveness of CIMT therapy on functional hand use in the impaired upper limb. the efficacy of this approach has not been established, in particular in relation to the adverse effects of prolonged immobilization of the normally developing upper limb.

Patterning

The concept of patterning is based on theories developed during the 1950's and 1960's by Fay, Delacato, and Doman. Patterning is based on the principle that typical development of the infant and child progresses through a well-established, pre-determined sequence's; with failure to typically complete one stage of development causing inhibition or impairment in the development of subsequent stages. Based on this principal they suggested that in children with Cerebral Palsy typical motor development can be facilitated by passively repeating and putting the child through the sequential steps of typical development, a process called patterning. Parents and other care givers are taught to carry out this patterning process at home but the approach is hugely labour intensive and time consuming as it requires multiple sessions every day. Although Patterning has been utilised for many years its use is now certainly controversial and the effectiveness has not been established. It is a very passive therapy, with little opportunity to encourage the child in their active involvement and its use in children with Cerebral Palsy is not recommended.

Therapeutic Interventions

Passive Stretching

It is a manual application for spastic muscles to relieve soft tissue tightness. Manual stretching may increase range of movements, reduce spasticity, or improve walking efficiency in children with spasticity. Stretch may be applied in a number of ways during neurological rehabilitation to achieve different effects. The types of stretching used include:

- Fast/Quick,
- Prolonged,
- Maintained.

When we look at the use of stretch for facilitation we employ a fast/quick stretch. The fast/quick stretch produce a relatively short lived contraction of the agonist muscle and short lived inhibition of the antagonist muscle which facilitates a muscle contraction. It achieves its effect via stimulation of the muscle spindle primary endings which results in reflex. Reflex facilitation of the muscle via the monosynaptic reflex arc.

The presence of increased tone can ultimately lead to joint contracture and changes in muscle length. When we look at the use of stretch to normalise tone and maintain soft tissue length we employ a slow, prolonged stretch to maintain or prevent loss of range of motion. While the effects are not entirely clear the prolonged stretch produces inhibition of muscle responses which may help in reducing hypertonus, e.g. Bobath's neuro-developmental technique, inhibitory splinting and casting technique. It appears to have an influence on both the neural components of muscle, via the Golgi Tendon Organs and Muscle Spindles, and the structural components in the long term, via the number and length of sarcomeres.

Muscle Immobilised Shortened Position = Loss of Sarcomeres and Increased Stiffness related to increase in connective tissue,

Muscle Immobilised Lengthened Position = Increase Sarcomeres

Studies in Mice show that a stretch of 30 mins daily will prevent the loss of sarcomeres in the connective tissue of an immobilised muscle, although the timescale in humans may not relate directly.

Passive stretching may be achieved through a number of methods which include:

- Manual Stretching: Prolonged manual stretch may be applied manually, using the effect of body weight and gravity or mechanically, using machine or splints.

Stretch should provide sufficient force to overcome hypertonicity and passively lengthen the muscle. Unlikely to provide sufficient stretch to cause change in a joint that already has contracture.

- Weight Bearing: Weight bearing has been reported to reduce contracture in the lower limb through use of Tilt-tables, and standing frames through a prolonged stretch. Angles are key to ensure the knees remain extend during the prolonged stretch as the force exerted on the knee can be quite high. Some research also challenges the assumption of the benefits of prolonged standing.

- Splinting: Splints and casts are external devices "Splints and casts are external devices designed to apply, distribute or remove forces to or from the body in a controlled manner to perform one or both basic functions of control of body motion and alteration or prevention in the shape of body tissue." Splinting can be used to produce low-force, long duration stretching although there is a dearth of evidence to support this. A wide range of splint have been used to influence swelling, resting posture, spasticity, active and passive ROM.

- Serial Casting: Serial casting is a common technique that is used and most effective in managing spasticity related contracture. Serial casting is a specialized technique to provide increased range of joint motion. The process involves a joint or joints that are tight which are immobilized with a semi-rigid, well-padded cast. Serial casting involves repeated applications of casts, typically every one to two weeks as range of motion is restored.

The duration of stretch to reduce both spasticity and to prevent contracture are not yet clear from the research and require further research to determine the most appropriate technique and duration to produce the required effect.

Static Weight-bearing Exercises

Stimulation of antigravity muscle strength, prevention of hip dislocation, reduction in spasticity and improvements in bone mineral density, self-confidence and motor function have all been achieved through the use of Static Weigh Bearing exercises such as Tilt-Table and Standing Frame.

Muscle Strengthening Exercises

It aims to increase the power of weak antagonist muscles and of the corresponding spastic agonists and to provide the functional benefits of strengthening in children with CP.

Functional Exercises

Training related to specific functional activities combining aerobic and anaerobic capacity and strength training in ambulatory children, has been shown to significantly improve overall physical fitness, the intensity of activities, and quality of life. Training programs on static bicycles or treadmill have been shown to be beneficial for gait and gross motor development but have not shown to have any impact on spasticity or abnormal movement patterns.

Body Weight Supported Treadmill Training

Stepping movements from Reflex Stepping Reactions are normally present in newborns and infants, before the infant starts to bear weight, stand and walk. Body Weight Supported Treadmill Training, is achieved through supporting the child in a harness on the treadmill in an upright posture limiting overall weight bearing, on a slow moving treadmill, eliciting the stepping movements. Treadmill training, thus allows development of stepping movements needed for ambulation. Studies using 3-4 sessions per week lasting for 3-4 months have shown improvement in lower extremity movements and gait patterns in children with cerebral palsy.

Electrical Stimulation

The goal of the electrical stimulation is to increase muscle strength and motor function. Electrical stimulation is provided by Transcutaneous Electrical Nerve Stimulation (TENS) Unit which is portable, non-invasive and can be used in the home-setting by parents or the patient. Neuromuscular Electrical Stimulation (NMES) involves application of transcutaneous electrical current that results in muscle contraction. NMES has been postulated to increase muscle strength by increasing the cross-sectional area of the muscle and by increased recruitment of type 2 muscle fibers. Functional Electrical Stimulation (FES) refers to the application of electrical stimulation during a given task or activity when a specific muscle is expected to be contracting. There is some evidence to support the use and effectiveness of NMES in children with Cerebral Palsy but found that many of the studies are limited by confounding variables including concomitant use of other therapies, wide variation in methods of application, heterogeneity of subjects, difficulty in measuring functional outcomes and lack of control subjects. proposes that neuromuscular and threshold electrical stimulation as a modality in Cerebral Palsy is used for strengthening the quadriceps muscles in ambulatory diplegic children with Cerebral Palsy, who have difficulty with specific resistive strength training.

Hippotherapy

Gross Motor Function including Muscle tone, Range of Movement, Balance, Coordination and Postural Control in children with CP have been shown to improve with Therapeutic horse-back riding which may reduce the degree of motor disability. Many none physical benefits may also be developed through enjoyment and providing a setting for increased social interaction, cognitive and psychosocial development. There is limited evidence available with two lower-quality trials on saddle riding on a horse found no between-group differences in muscle symmetry or in any of the seven different outcome measures, except on a sub-item of grasping.

State of the Evidence

Novak et al have developed a chart based on their Systamatic Study, which looked at the State of the Evidence in relation to Interventions for the management of children with Cerebral Palsy, to assist with comparative clinical decision-making amongst intervention options for the same desired outcome. They mapped the interventions using bubble charts, with the the size of the circle correlated to the volume of published evidence.

The circle size was calculated using:

- Number of published papers on the topic.

- Total score for the level of evidence (calculated by reverse coding of the Oxford Levels of Evidence, i.e. expert opinion=1, randomized controlled trial [RCT] = 5).

- Location of the circle on the Y-Axis of the graph corresponds to the GRADE System Rating.

- Colour of the circle correlates to the Evidence Alert System.

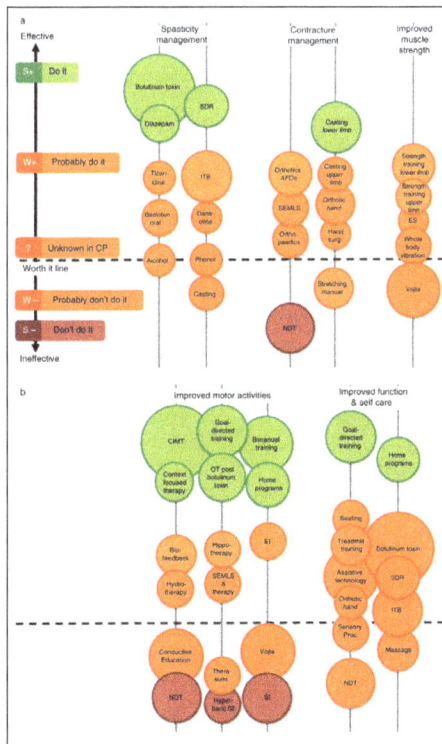

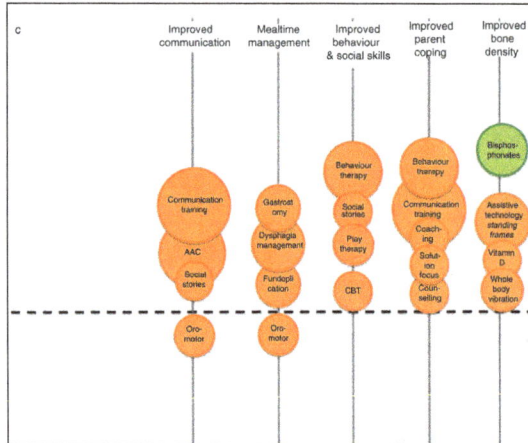

Pediatric Muscular Dystrophies

Muscular dystrophy (MD) is a broad term that describes a genetic (inherited) disorder of the muscles. Muscular dystrophy causes the muscles in the body to become very weak. The muscles break down and are replaced with fatty deposits over time.

Other health problems commonly associated with muscular dystrophy include the following:

- Heart problems.

- Scoliosis: A lateral, or sideways, curvature and rotation of the back bones (vertebrae), giving the appearance that the person is leaning to one side.

- Obesity.

The most common forms of muscular dystrophy are Duchenne muscular dystrophy (DMD) and Becker muscular dystrophy. The two forms are very similar, but Becker muscular dystrophy is less severe than DMD. Girls are rarely affected by either of these two forms of muscular dystrophy.

Causes of Muscular Dystroph

Duchenne muscular dystrophy is a genetic disease which means it is inherited. Our genes determine our traits, such as eye color and blood type. Genes are contained in the cells of our bodies on stick-like structures called chromosomes. There are normally 46 chromosomes in each cell of our body, or 23 pairs. The first 22 pairs are shared in common between males and females, while the last pair determine gender and are called the sex chromosome pair: females have two X chromosomes, while males have one X and one Y chromosome.

Duchenne muscular dystrophy is caused by an X-linked recessive gene. "X-linked" means that the gene causing the trait or the disorder is located on the X chromosome. Genes on the X chromosome can be recessive or dominant, and their expression in females and males is not the same because the genes on the Y chromosome do not exactly pair up with the genes on the X. X-linked recessive genes are expressed in females only if there are two copies of the gene (one on each X chromosome). However, for males there only needs to be one copy of an X-linked recessive gene in order for the trait or disorder to be expressed. For example, a woman can carry a recessive gene on one of the X chromosomes unknowingly, and pass it on to a son, who will express the trait or disease.

Symptoms of Muscular Dystrophy

Muscular dystrophy is usually diagnosed in children between 3 and 6 years of age. Early signs of the illness include a delay in walking, difficulty rising from a sitting or lying position, and frequent falling, with weakness typically affecting the shoulder and pelvic muscle as one of the initial symptoms. The following are the most common symptoms of muscular dystrophy. However, each child may experience symptoms differently. Symptoms may include:

- Clumsy movement,

- Difficulty climbing stairs,

- Frequently trips and falls,

- Unable to jump or hop normally,

- Tip toe walking,

- Leg pain,

- Facial weakness,

- Inability to close eyes or whistle,

- Shoulder and arm weakness.

A clinical characteristic for Duchenne muscular dystrophy (DMD) is Gowers' sign. Children with Duchenne muscular dystrophy find it very hard to get up from a sitting or lying position on the floor. They first pull up to their hands and knees. The child walks his or her hands up their legs to brace themselves as they rise to a standing position.

In addition, children with muscular dystrophy often have very large calves due to the large amounts of fatty deposits that are replacing muscle.

The symptoms of muscular dystrophy may resemble other conditions or medical problems. Always consult your child's doctor for a diagnosis.

Diagnosis of Muscular Dystrophy

The diagnosis of muscular dystrophy is made with a physical examination and diagnostic testing by your child's physician. During the examination, your child's doctor obtains a complete prenatal and birth history of the child and asks if other family members are known to have muscular dystrophy.

Diagnostic tests for muscular dystrophy may include:

- Blood tests: These include genetic blood tests.

- Muscle biopsy: The primary test used to confirm diagnosis. A small sample of muscle tissue is taken and examined under a microscope.

- Electromyogram (EMG): A test to check if the muscle weakness is a result of destruction of muscle tissue rather than nerve damage.

- Electrocardiogram (ECG or EKG): A test that records the electrical activity of the heart, shows abnormal rhythms (arrhythmias or dysrhythmias), and detects heart muscle damage.

Treatment for Muscular Dystrophy

Specific treatment for muscular dystrophy will be determined by your child's doctor based on:

- Your child's age, overall health, and medical history.

- The extent of the condition.

- The type of condition.

- Your child's tolerance for specific medications, procedures, or therapies.

- Expectations for the course of the condition.

- Your opinion or preference.

To date, there is no known treatment, medicine, or surgery that will cure muscular dystrophy, or stop the muscles from weakening. The goal of treatment is to prevent deformity and allow the child to function as independently as possible.

Since muscular dystrophy is a life-long condition that is not correctable, management includes focusing on preventing or minimizing deformities and maximizing the child's functional ability at home and in the community.

Management of muscular dystrophy is either nonsurgical or surgical. Nonsurgical interventions may include:

- Physical therapy.

- Positioning aids used to help the child sit, lie, or stand.

- Braces and splints used to prevent deformity, promote support, or provide protection.

- Medications.

- Nutritional counselling.

- Psychological counselling.

Surgical interventions may be considered to manage the following conditions:

- Scoliosis (a sideways curvature of the back bones) associated with muscular dystrophy.

- Maintaining the child's ability to sit or stand.

Long-term Outlook for a Child with Muscular Dystrophy

Muscular dystrophy is a progressive condition that needs life-long management to prevent deformity and complications. Walking and sitting often becomes more difficult as the child grows. Usually by the age of 12, the child needs a wheelchair because the leg muscles are too weak to work. Heart or lung problems often occur by the late teenage years or into the early 20s.

The interdisciplinary health care team will work with your family to improve your child's functional outcomes and to provide support as you learn to care for your child's needs.

Rehabilitation Management

DMD is characterized by well-known patterns of progressive muscle degeneration and weakness, postural compensations, risk of progressive contracture and deformity, and functional losses resulting from dystrophin deficiency. The natural history of DMD has changed over the years with more comprehensive medical and therapeutic management, the use of glucocorticoids, and the advent of emerging disease-modifying treatments.

These advances have resulted in prolonged ambulation, decreases and/or delays in the development of severe contracture and deformity (including scoliosis), improved cardiorespiratory status, and prolonged function into adulthood. Patients have been supported by advancing adaptive equipment, assistive technology, and "smart" technology, all of which promise ever-increasing participation in adulthood.

Assessment

Multidisciplinary assessment across the International Classification of Functioning, Disability, and Health and care continuum remains important in guiding rehabilitation interventions. Assessment tools recommended in the original (2010) Care Considerations remain supported and expanded via newly developed tools. Impairment-level measures include passive ranges of motion (ROM) and the assessment of alignment and posture, which is critical in monitoring the success of musculoskeletal management and identifying needs for additional physical therapy (PT), occupational therapy (OT), orthotic intervention, serial casting, seating system modification, supported standing, and adaptive equipment. Standardized functional assessments for DMD have been expanded with the establishment of validity, reliability, predictive potential, and minimal clinically important differences, These assessments should be used across the life span Use of the same measures over time, including new assessments as appropriate, is recommended to monitor change and support anticipatory management. Measurement of pain, fatigue, disability, participation, quality of life, and patient-reported outcomes are important as is the increasing use of activity monitoring. Occupational therapist assessment of learning, attentional, and sensory processing differences, fine motor function, and activities of daily living (ADL) should begin early, guiding intervention and optimizing success. Multidisciplinary assessment across the International Classification of Functioning, Disability, and Health should occur at least every 6 months, with more frequent assessment being triggered by concern, change in status, or specific needs as supported by professional standards of care.

Orthotic Intervention, Splints, and/or Adaptive Equipment for Stretching:

- AFOs for stretching:
    - Modified leaf-spring AFOs (lighter weight, less cumbersome, allow for some movement) for use at night or during daytime periods when not walking.
    - Articulating AFOs may offer more movement for increased tolerance at night, but can be bulkier.
    - Adjustable-angle AFOs to try to gain increased range (a little bulkier) for use at night or during daytime periods when not walking.
    - Modular (3-piece) AFOs for use in combinations of night use and/or daytime use in nonambulatory stages.
    - Ankle height (supramalleolar during the day to maintain medial-lateral alignment if 90° maintained by footrest).
    - Taller AFO component to prevent plantar flexor tightness; may be rigid, flexible, or articulating (hinged) depending on need, tolerance, and preference.

- Inner liner for comfort (can be important in any AFO).

- Serial casting.

- Knee extension splints.

- KAFOs (or "long leg braces").

- Stander and stand-and-drive motorized wheelchair.

- Hand and wrist splints to maintain length in long wrist and finger flexors.

- Stretching gloves to maintain length in finger extensors.

- Oval-8 finger splints to prevent hyperextension at proximal interphalangeal joint.

Intervention

Comprehensive, anticipatory, preventive rehabilitation management is focused on protecting fragile muscles; preserving and maintaining optimal strength; minimizing the progression of weakness when possible; preventing and minimizing progressive contracture and deformity; supporting optimal cardiorespiratory care and function; optimizing energy efficiency and energy conservation; providing adaptive equipment and assistive technology; maintaining skin integrity; preventing and minimizing pain; supporting function, functional independence, and participation at school, work, and in family and social life; and optimizing quality of life.

A multidisciplinary rehabilitation team is required that includes physicians, physical therapists, occupational therapists, speech-language pathologists, orthotists, and providers of durable medical equipment who coordinate with those in pulmonary medicine, orthopedics, cardiology, neurology, genetics, social work, psychology, endocrinology, nutrition, and gastroenterology. Direct skilled PT, OT, and speech-language therapy, based on individual assessment, are provided in outpatient, home, and school settings and in inpatient settings during hospitalizations and should be continued throughout adulthood.

Musculoskeletal Management (Prevention of Contracture and Deformity)

Anticipatory preventive musculoskeletal management is focused on preserving muscle extensibility, joint mobility, and symmetry to prevent and minimize contracture and deformity and should be a component of care at all stages. Joint contractures and diminished muscle extensibility in DMD result from interacting factors, including a lack of full active joint ROM, static positioning, and imbalanced muscle weakness across joints. Fibrotic changes in the muscle begin with early fibrosis in the newborn period, revealing the importance of early preventive management of muscle flexibility and extensibility. Effective maintenance of joint ROM, muscle extensibility, and prevention of contracture and deformity requires multiple coordinated interventions, including active and active-assisted elongation; daily passive stretching of joints, muscles, and soft tissues at risk for tightness and those identified via assessment; prolonged elongation; and support of optimal positioning throughout the day with splinting, orthotic intervention, standing devices, custom seating in mobility devices, and adaptive equipment.

PT and OT Interventions for Musculoskeletal Management

Stretching to prevent and minimize contractures should be done a minimum of 4 to 6 days per week for joints and muscle groups known to be at risk for hypoextensibility and those identified via assessment. When stretching, providers should include manual therapy techniques, avoid the elicitation of pain, and establish a preventative stretching program before decreases in passive ROM occur, with direct PT and OT accompanied by support of optimal positioning and the use of splinting and orthotic intervention, custom seating systems, supported standing, and adaptive equipment. Preventive stretching of lower extremities (LEs) should be initiated early in the ambulatory phase and continued through adulthood. Preventive stretching of upper extremities (UEs) and the neck becomes increasingly important in nonambulatory stages and throughout adulthood. Increased risk areas for contracture and deformity in adults with DMD necessitate detailed assessment and intervention over time. The maintenance of chest wall mobility is important in respiratory management and the prevention of scoliosis. Local care should be augmented by guidance from specialists every 4 to 6 months.

Orthotic Intervention and Adaptive Equipment for Musculoskeletal Management

The prevention of contractures and deformity requires preventive splinting and orthotic intervention, positioning, supported standing programs, and the use of adaptive equipment and assistive technology in addition to manual stretching programs.

Orthoses

Resting or stretching ankle-foot orthoses (AFOs) are necessary, with nighttime use having been shown to prevent and minimize progressive plantarflexion contractures, and are appropriate throughout life. AFOs should be custom molded, fabricated for comfort and optimum foot-ankle alignment. They are typically best tolerated if started preventively at young ages. Blanket lifter bars may ease bed mobility, increasing tolerance of nighttime AFO use. If nighttime tolerance cannot be achieved, the use of stretching AFOs during nonambulatory portions of the day is encouraged. Daytime AFO use can be appropriate for full-time wheelchair users, extending into adulthood. Lower-profile orthoses may be considered for full-time wheelchair users to control plantar varus if adequate medial-lateral positioning is maintained and adequate dorsiflexion is supported by wheelchair footrests. Knee-ankle-foot orthoses (KAFOs) (eg, long leg braces or calipers) for support-ed standing, limited ambulation for therapeutic purposes, and the prevention of contrac-ture and deformity in late-ambulatory and early nonambulatory stages evolving and may not be tolerated at night. Adjustable knee extension splints can be considered for assis-tance in maintaining knee extension range in nonambulatory individuals. Comfortable support of neutral LE positioning in bed helps minimize contracture. The use of resting hand splints, stretching gloves, and oval-8 finger splints is appropriate, continuing into adulthood for stabilization, support, and musculoskeletal management.

Standing Devices

Supported standing devices for individuals with no or mild LE contractures are nec-essary for late-ambulatory and early nonambulatory stages, including standers and stand-and-drive motorized wheelchairs, extending benefits previously reported with the use of KAFOs. Supported standing for prolonged passive elongation of LE mus-culature should be considered when standing and walking in good alignment become difficult. The importance of initiating the preventive use of supported standing be-fore the development of contractures should be emphasized. Many advocate for the continued use of supported standing devices and a powered stand-and-drive motor-ized wheelchair into late-nonambulatory stages and throughout adulthood if contrac-tures do not limit positioning and if devices are tolerated. Motorized stand-and-drive wheelchairs obviate the need for transfers to use supported standing, decreasing the risk of falls and increasing the number of hours per day of functional, comfortable, supported standing.

Serial Casting

Serial casting can be considered when stretching and orthotic use have not maintained adequate ROM and when surgery is not preferred or chosen. Serial casting for ambula-tory individuals is used only if ambulation remains possible while casted with sufficient quadriceps strength to avoid compromising ambulation and losing function. In nonam-bulatory individuals, the risk of functional loss is less, but cast weight may compromise transfers, necessitating lift use, and may be contraindicated with severe contractures. Skin integrity and osteoporosis must also be considered. An experienced team is re-quired for the successful use of serial casting.

KAFOs

The prolongation of ambulation for 2 to 4 years has historically been reported with KAFOs, with or without accompanying LE surgery, and associated with decreases in scoliosis and LE contracture, although with contextual qualifications, including indi-vidual, family, and team preferences, and greater success with experienced teams and in the absence of obesity. Individuals with DMD, who are now walking longer with glucocorticoids even without KAFOs, have differing height and body configurations at ambulation loss (decreased height, increased BMI, and increased relative hip abduction and/or external rotation versus spinal extension). These differences present challenges in wearing KAFOs, including an increased risk of fracture as a result of a higher risk of falls. Moreover, technological options, including increasingly routine use of stand-and-drive motorized wheelchairs, may be more common than KAFOs to maintain supported standing mobility. However, reports of KAFO use with glucocorticoids prolonging ambulation to even older ages, family satisfaction in spite of challenges, and situations in which KAFOs are the only means of supported standing suggest that KAFOs continue to be an appropriate option in some contexts. Rapidly advancing technology in robotics offers potentially improved future options. KAFO use should be viewed as therapeutic rather than functional, with care taken to support safety to minimize the risk of falls, and not used exclusive of motorized mobility, which is typically provided simultaneously or earlier for safe, optimal, functional independence; mobility; and participation in all settings.

Falls and Fracture Prevention and Management

Physical therapist collaboration with those in orthopedics to prevent falls and fractures and maintain or regain ambulation after a long bone fracture is increasingly emphasized. Extended ambulatory capacity, coupled with the risk of low-trauma fractures, increases the importance of fall prevention, including fall risk assessment across settings, pool shoes for fall prevention when walking on slippery surfaces, and the early use of lift and transfer equipment, especially in bathrooms, where transfer challenges compromise safety. Rapid appropriate team management of long bone fractures with associated rehabilitation is essential and may include the temporary use of assistive devices and other types of support to minimize the risk of loss of ambulation and prevent accelerated contracture and deformity.

Learning, Attentional and Sensory Processing Issues

OT is important for early assessment and intervention for learning, attentional, and sensory processing issues, which are increasingly understood as being important in DMD.

Areas for Specialized OT Assessment and Intervention:

- Learning differences (specific differences in DMD are increasingly identified, including differences between verbal and performance IQ and differences in verbal memory, dyslexia, dyscalculia, and dysgraphia).
- Attentional issues.
- Sensory processing issues.
- Fine motor.

- ADL.

- Computer access.

- Assistive technology.

- Swallowing and oral motor dysfunction.

- Planning for academics and vocation in transition to adulthood.

Exercise and Activity Levels

Physical therapists prescribe, monitor, and guide exercise in DMD on the basis of understanding potential effects of activity and exercise on dystrophin-deficient muscle. Concern about exercise hastening the progression of weakness in DMD is longstanding based on pathophysiology, including the risks of contraction-induced muscle injury and exercise-induced structural damage related to strength, the duration of contraction, and the load imposed. Other concerns include nitric oxide synthase dysfunction leading to increased ischemia during exercise and cardiac concerns, including a lack of correlation between skeletal and cardiac muscle involvement with moderately to severely reduced exercise capacity, as measured by cardiopulmonary exercise testing, even in the presence of normal or mildly impaired gross motor function and capacity. The balance between beneficial versus harmful effects of muscle activity are not fully understood. Certain amounts of muscle activity are assumed to be beneficial in preventing disuse atrophy, maintaining residual strength, providing or maintaining potential trophic influences of active movement, and maintaining functional status and flexibility, but eccentric muscle activity and maximal- or high-resistance exercise are believed to be detrimental and inappropriate across the life span because of potential contraction-induced muscle-fiber injury. Specifics regarding the optimal type, frequency, and intensity of exercise in DMD are not definitively known. Participation in regular, gentle aerobic functional activity, such as aquatics, cycling, and safe recreation-based activity, is recommended by some, especially early in the course of the disease, when residual strength is higher, with an emphasis on moderation, lower-duration activity, support of self-initiated rests, and the avoidance of overexertion and overwork weakness. Aquatics, with potential benefits for aerobic-conditioning respiratory exercise and support of gravity-minimized movement, is highly recommended for the early ambulatory through nonambulatory stages and into adulthood as long as it is medically safe. Cycling is recommended as a submaximal aerobic form of activity, with benefits of assisted cycling recently reported.

Fibrosis (beginning in the newborn period, before extensive cell necrosis), the proliferation of connective tissue, and increased stiffness, increases loads (resistance) against which muscles must work, further taxing contractile units and potentially contributing to ischemia and vascular and structural impediments to regeneration. The role of active movement, positive or negative, on the fibrotic process and vascularity is not clear.

Individualized assessment and monitoring of activity levels is important. Significant muscle pain or myoglobinuria in the 24-hour period after a specific activity is a sign of overexertion and contraction-induced injury, and if it occurs, the activity should be modified.

Cardiac concerns regarding exercise include cardiomyopathy and/or arrhythmias, abnormalities of calcium regulation, and cardiac wall movement fibrosis fatty infiltration; and conduction abnormalities. These typically progress to dilated cardiomyopathy with arrhythmias, including ventricular tachycardia. Early cardiac involvement can be present even before overt clinical manifestations. Symptoms may not present until cardiac involvement is more advanced because of limited physical activity and a lack of correlation between cardiac and skeletal muscle involvement, supporting caution in prescribing exercise for individuals with dystrophinopathies, who appear likely to have a reduced exercise capacity even when functioning well. Individuals with DMD should have early referral to cardiology for the identification and preventive management of cardiomyopathy.

Assistive and Adaptive Devices for Function

AFOs are not typically indicated for use during ambulation because they tend to limit the compensatory movements needed for efficient ambulation, add weight that can compromise ambulation, and make it difficult to rise from the floor and climb stairs. During the late-ambulatory stage, KAFOs with locked knees can prolong ambulation but with use decreased.

During the early ambulatory stage, lightweight manual mobility devices are appropriate for pushing the child on occasions when long-distance mobility demands exceed endurance. In the late-ambulatory stage and early nonambulatory stages, an ultralightweight manual wheelchair with custom seating to support spinal symmetry and LE alignment and swing-away footrests is necessary and may be used in situations without access or transport for motorized mobility. A variety of motorized mobility devices, including standing mobility devices, may be used intermittently for energy conservation and independent long-distance mobility by individuals who continue to walk.

As functional community ambulation becomes more difficult, a motorized wheelchair is advocated. Custom seating and power-positioning components for the initial motorized wheelchair are important standards of care, with power stand-and-drive having been shown to be used more successfully if initiated before the development of contracture and deformity. Custom seating for safety, support of optimal posture, and the prevention of contracture and deformity includes a solid seat with hip guides and a pressure relief cushion; a solid planar back with rigid lateral trunk supports; flip-down, swing-away, or removable knee adductors; and a headrest. Facial components on headrests may be needed in older individuals for adequate head support and symmetry. Swing-away or flip-up footrests facilitate transfers. Power-positioning components include power tilt and recline, power stand-and-drive, power-adjustable seat height, and separately elevating power-elevating leg rests. Elbow supports may be needed for UE support that keeps the hand on the joystick during position changes and on rough terrain. Retractable, swing-away joystick hardware and trays may be needed for access. Lights and blinkers are required for safety in evening community mobility. Ventilator holders are needed for those using ventilatory support.

Assistive Technology

Referral to assistive technology (AT) specialists should be considered whenever function, independence, and participation are compromised, and is necessary when UE weakness affects reach, fine motor skills, and ADL. AT is helpful in optimizing fine motor skills, enhancing strategies for independence in ADL, and improving access to alternative computer, mobility, or environmental control. Simple adaptations supporting UE function include elevated lap trays and/or desks, adaptive straws, a hands-free water pouch, and/or turntables if the hand cannot be brought to the mouth or if biceps strength is <3 in 5. More advanced AT options include motorized and nonmotorized mobile arm supports (considered at Brooke Upper Extremity Scale score ≥2), robotics, miniature-proportional joysticks, microswitches, Bluetooth capabilities, software and applications for computers, fall detection systems with built-in Global Positioning System detection, voice activation and texting systems on smartphones and tablets, and "smart home systems" that are able to interface with motorized wheelchairs. Key pinch, microswitches, mouth call buttons, and monitoring systems are considered if hand or voice weakness precludes the use of standard call buttons. Adaptive equipment for the support of ADL, safety, and the maintenance of skin integrity include power-adjustable beds with pressure-relieving mattresses; bathing and toileting equipment; lift and/or transfer devices, including hydraulic and motorized patient lifts; ceiling lifts (hoists); slide sheets; and environmental control options.

AT assessment and intervention are focused on optimizing function and participation across the life span, which are particularly important during transitions between functional levels and transitioning into adulthood.

Extended ambulation, the importance of energy conservation for muscle preservation and function, and increased independence into adulthood require expanded technology for mobility, a greater variety of choices for different situations, and increased AT options for mobility, driving, and community access that are instrumental in participation, employment, and avoidance of social isolation. Vehicle adaptations increase options for community access, and adapted controls may allow for independent vehicle driving. Skill development via accessible public transportation, OT driving evaluation, and future driverless cars promise ongoing increases in independence.

The early development of independent decision-making and respectful and responsible delegation skills in children with DMD, supported by the use of AT, self-advocacy skills, the hiring and directing of aides, the use of service animals, and social participation foster transitions to independent adult function.

Funding for the support of AT and support services is critical, as is the education of families about funding opportunities, including private insurance, Medicaid, Medicaid Waiver programs, Medicare, Independent Living, Vocational Rehabilitation, Supplemental Security Income, Achieving a Better Life Experience accounts, and other funding sources, which vary depending on the country, state, and local environment.

Pain Management

Pain, which is considered the fifth vital sign, is important to assess in all individuals with DMD across the life span. A more uniform assessment of pain, however, does not always lead to successful management of pain, which is an important priority in transitions to adulthood and the management of DMD in adulthood. Pain of varying types and intensities may occur in DMD. Effective pain management requires an accurate determination of the cause and may require comprehensive team management. Postural correction, orthotic intervention, PT, adaptive equipment, assistive technology, and pharmacological interventions may all be required. Adaptive equipment and assistive technology should be used to emphasize the prevention and management of pain and optimize comfortable function and movement with transfer, bathing, and toileting equipment. Power-positioning components offering positional support and change, weight shift, and pressure relief on motorized wheelchairs and beds can be used as needed to maintain skin integrity and pain prevention or relief. Providers of pharmacological interventions must consider possible interactions with other medications (e.g, steroids and non-steroidal anti-inflammatory drugs) and side effects, particularly those that might negatively affect cardiac or respiratory function. Rarely, orthopedic intervention might be indicated for intractable pain that is amenable to surgery. Back pain, especially if the patient is receiving glucocorticoids, is an indication for careful assessment for vertebral fractures.

Key Anticipatory Discussions for Rehabilitation

Key anticipatory discussions should occur before a time of crisis in each of the following areas. Care team members can reassure the patient and family that rather than being evidence of disease progression, these issues provide opportunities to discuss options for optimizing management:

- Plans for when stairclimbing becomes difficult.

- Continuum of options for energy conservation and safe, functional, independent mobility and participation in all settings.

- Fall risk assessment and prevention.

- Fracture management.

- Initiating supported standing.

- Transfers and/or access at home, at school, at work, and in the community.

- Consideration of KAFO use.

- Spine surgery.

- Strategies for optimizing ADL and self-feeding compromised by UE weakness or spine fusion.

- Noninvasive ventilation and tracheostomy.

As disease-modifying treatments become available, questions will emerge regarding potential increases in exercise capacity and muscle recovery, optimizing potential benefit versus damage from specific types, durations, and frequency of exercise. Robotics and AT advances are anticipated to provide ever increasing functional independence, capacity for participation, and successful musculoskeletal management, and it will be important to explore ways that these developments can be used to benefit individuals with DMD.

Pediatric Rehabilitation Medicine

Pediatric rehabilitation medicine (PRM) is the subspecialty that uses an interdisciplinary approach to address the prevention, diagnosis, treatment, and management of congenital and childhood-onset physical impairments including related or secondary medical, physical, functional, psychosocial, cognitive, and vocational limitations or conditions, with an understanding of the life course of disability. Childhood disability is on the rise. Children with disabilities have more health care needs and more unmet needs for health services. As a field, pediatric rehabilitation medicine (PRM) plays a vital role in the care of these children. This is true now more than ever because of the increasing advances in lifesaving treatments and the growth of childhood chronic conditions, of which many are associated with disabilities.

Pediatric Rehabilitation Methods

Occupational Therapy

Occupational therapists evaluate a child's current skills for typical daily activities and then compare those to what is age appropriate. The occupational therapists will then help the child develop fine motor skills, sensory motor skills, and visual motor skills that children need to socialize appropriately. Children with spina bifida, burns, learning problems, birth defects, traumatic injuries, juvenile rheumatoid arthritis, and many other medical conditions can benefit from occupational therapy.

Some methods include using weighted vests, Neuro-Developmental Treatment (NDT), motor learning theories, therapeutic listening, assistive technology, or simply incorporating play more often. Occupational therapists often try new techniques and methods to enhance a child's skills for playing, academic performance, socializing, and other daily activities.

Physical Therapy

To improve strength, posture, range of motion, flexibility, movement patterns, or balance for a child, including for spine injury rehabilitation, physical therapy can be instrumental. Children with developmental delays, genetic disorders, muscle coordination concerns, birth defects, and orthopedic disabilities, among many other conditions, can all benefit from physical therapy. Movement is key in academic and social settings, so by improving children's movement abilities through physical therapy, everything else will be affected as well.

Methods include Neuro-Developmental Treatment (NDT), strength training, endurance training, use of orthotics, and kinesiotaping, among others. Aquatic (water) therapy and equine (horse) therapy are two fun, unique, and effective forms of pediatric physical therapy. Hippotherapy (physical therapy that uses the movement of a horse) research indicates causation between the therapy and improved muscle symmetry in children with spastic cerebral palsy. Research also show improvements among children who regularly participate in aquatic therapy.

Speech-language Therapy

Communication, obviously, is another common concern and can be addressed with therapy. Speech-language pathologists can help children understand and access the tools they need to communicate effectively. Whether this is part of brain injury rehabilitation or is due to a preexisting condition, a speech-language pathologist can help a child with both verbal and non-verbal language. They can also help feeding and swallowing in infants and children.

Neuro-Developmental Treatment (NDT) is once again a common method. Other methods include the Sequential Oral Sensory (SOS) Approach to Feeding and specialized skills for assessing and treating infants. Studies show that speech-language therapy is extremely useful for children with phonological or vocabulary difficulties.

Pediatric Neurorehabilitation Medicine

The application of rehabilitation extends far beyond the bounds of traditional medicine since one of its chief aims is to protect or restore personal and social identity.

Neurorehabilitation therefore encompasses two distinct, but overlapping, concepts. The first is that neurorehabilitation is a medical subspecialty that treats patients with disabling (and often chronic) diseases of the central and peripheral nervous system. So defined, neurorehabilitation translates into the active process designed to reduce the effects of a primary neurological condition on performance of activities in daily life. A second aspect stresses the specific therapeutic modalities that are implemented to overcome or improve any neurological impairment that interferes with daily life. Both aspects clearly have practical implications for neurorehabilitation as it is carried out in children.

The principles, goals, and challenges of both pediatric neurorehabilitation and rehabilitation in general are best understood in the context of the International Classification of Functioning, Disability and Health, which replaces the previous scheme entitled the International Classification of Impairments, Disabilities and Handicaps. As originally defined by the World Health Organization, impairment is the loss or abnormality of physiologic, psychologic, or anatomic structure or function, while disability, the lack of ability or restricted ability to perform a functional task, is very dependent upon the individual's environment. Thus, one of the ways in which neurorehabilitation can be carried out is to modify or adapt the environment. Appropriate neurorehabilitation of disability in childhood must be predicated upon a clear understanding of normal development, as well as the ramifications of abnormal development. Finally, it must be recognized that disability does not flow solely or directly from the type and degree of impairment. Instead, disability is best viewed as a three-dimensional construct, consisting of impairment, activity limitations, and participation restrictions. Each dimension is the result of interaction between the biologic features intrinsic to the individual's medical condition and the child's physical and social environment.

The concept of dependency also plays a fundamental role in medical rehabilitation. Dependency is more readily quantifiable than disability, and degree of dependency is a critical element in the cost of on-going medical and rehabilitation care, as well as in eventual quality of life. While a variety of scales have been developed to measure a patient's potential autonomy, or conversely, the burden imposed on a caregiver, use in pediatric patients is limited because of the inter-related issues of anticipated development and maturation, the WeeFIM (Functional Independence Measure) is a very useful rehabilitation tool.

The disablement/dependency paradigm in pediatric neurorehabilitation emphasizes movement towards appropriate functional outcomes, as well as diagnosis, and thus is more informative than traditional neurodiagnostic categories. There also appear to be other distinct advantages to conceptualizing neurorehabilitation in this manner. First, therapeutic interventions and treatment modalities should be based primarily on the disablement and resultant activity limitations, as opposed to the underlying pathologic process producing the impairment. In practical terms, this means that rehabilitation techniques often may be transferred successfully from one child to another despite differences in their primary neurological diagnosis. Similarly, the process of neurorehabilitation logically involves a multidisciplinary team, comprised of physicians, nurses, therapists, and other healthcare professionals, who work in collaboration with the patient and the patient's family. Finally, the paradigm provides a framework for patients that can be expanded to encompass all of the multifaceted aspects of neurorehabilitation inherent in the practice of child neurology. For example, the paradigm works just as well in describing an adolescent with seizures (impairment) who is prohibited from driving an automobile (disablement) and thus relies on his parents for rides (dependency), as it does for a child with a lower thoracic spinal cord injury causing paralysis of the legs and thus a limited capacity to ambulate. In both cases, there are resultant activity limitations that will affect social life and future employment opportunities.

Mechanisms Underlying Functional Recovery in the Nervous System

Implicit in any consideration of the rehabilitation process is the recognition that the potential for recovery of function exists. The degree of recovery following injury to the nervous system is variable but rarely complete. None the less, a better understanding of the cellular and molecular bases of neuronal dysfunction, as well as the potential mechanisms by which recovery of function occurs, is the framework upon which development of any pediatric neurorehabilitation program must rest. Since each proposed mechanism of recovery follows a different time course, the implications are very important in defining an appropriate therapy program.

Mechanisms regarding potential recovery of neurological function are, at best, poorly understood. However, several general conclusions, based upon an increasing amount of scientific evidence, can be drawn. First, significant capabilities of biologic modification in response to injury and developmental aberrations exist within the nervous system. The potential mechanisms by which the nervous system can respond to injury are exceedingly varied and more dynamic than suggested by prior studies. Finally, meaningful recovery of function continues for an extended period of time, one that is longer than previously recognized. These findings stand in contrast to former beliefs that recovery essentially was a biphasic process, in that any improvement that occurred within the first few months following an injury was felt to be due to reversibility of factors affecting dysfunctional, as opposed to dead, tissue. Improvement in functional capabilities at later time periods was attributed to nonphysiologic factors, such as learning and behavior modification. Presently, however, there is strong evidence that changes in neuronal circuitry, as opposed to psychologic factors, mediate recovery of function. The level of scientific information does not allow us to separate out one set of factors from another. Concerning acquired injury to the central nervous system (CNS), it is appropriate to acknowledge that there is ongoing debate concerning the relative contributions of biological healing and learned adaptations to the process of functional recovery.

Resolution of Temporary Dysfunction

The mechanisms underlying recovery of function that occurs within the hours to days following injury to the nervous system most likely relate to resolution of temporary dysfunction in areas of the brain that have not been damaged irreversibly. Potential factors causing transient functional impairment include mild tissue hypoxia, elevated intracranial pressure, edema (both cytotoxic and vasogenic), small contusions and/or focal hematomas, and reversible depression of metabolic and enzymatic activity in areas of the nervous system remote from the primary injury. Clinical and experimental evidence supports each of the first four factors described above. Furthermore, focal brain injury can result in depression of metabolic activity in noncontiguous brain areas, as a result of a decrease in transmitter synthesizing enzymes in regions of damage. In a similar fashion, the concept of "diaschisis" has evolved, as a form of neural shock in which uninvolved areas of the brain are rendered temporarily nonfunctional when deprived of appropriate input from a remote area of injured brain. Recovery of function presumably transpires as a result of increased neurotransmitter synthesis, or more likely, elevated production of neurotransmitter receptors. Some portion of early recovery (12–24 hours lasting up to a week) in humans following brain injury may relate to resolution of similar metabolic derangements.

Reorganization of Neuronal Connections

Another potential mechanism by which recovery may occur following nervous system injury is via modification of active neural connections. Three specific modifications of neural connections – axonal regeneration, axon retraction, and collateral sprouting – have been touted as the most promising examples of reorganizational mechanisms in the nervous system. Axonal regeneration, the process by which damaged axons regrow to their normal target, serves as a dominant process of recovery in the peripheral nervous system. Whether it plays any significant role in the restoration of brain function in humans is debatable, since regeneration in the mammalian CNS rarely has been documented, and then only under highly artificial conditions. Other mechanisms by which neuronal reorganization transpires include axon retraction and the associated process of pruning of synapses in the developing brain. In the early stages of development, certain axons project branches that ultimately are destined to be retracted at a later time. Similarly, maturation of the cerebral cortex in children in early postnatal life is characterized by an initial proliferation of synapse formation, followed later by activity-dependent pruning of excessive synapses.

The duration of this dynamic change in synaptic number varies between specific regions of cortex, but in the frontal lobe, synaptic thickening still is evident well into teenage years. The time course of programmed retraction of axon collaterals, although less well established, likely also is confined to early development. Research now indicates that this normal retraction process may not occur if nervous system injury is sustained early on, thus providing a mechanism for retention of function. For example, positron emission tomographic (PET) and functional magnetic resonance imaging (fMRI) studies have demonstrated that, following hemispherectomy for refractory childhood epilepsy, recovery of motor function in the leg contralateral to the surgery is associated with enhanced activation of the ipsilateral hemisphere, presumably via persistent ipsilateral corticospinal tracts. However, following stroke, neuronal activity in the cortex opposite the side of damage actually correlates with reduced functional recovery.

Multiple brain activation paradigms in stroke patients have revealed that functional improvement largely is dependent on cortical reorganization strategies within brain connected with or adjacent to the region of injury. The mechanism primarily responsible for this type of recovery is collateral sprouting, also termed reactive synaptogenesis. This process involves the axonal outgrowth from undamaged neurons and the establishment of synaptic contact at sites vacated by degenerating or dying neurons. Collateral sprouting typically is confined to brain regions normally innervated by nerve cells sharing common features with the injured neurons. Additionally, the axonal growth cones respect certain anatomic boundaries and, thus, their movement is not into novel nervous system domains. Collateral sprouting appears to be greatly influenced by growth and apoptotic factors. Thus, it is not surprising that the magnitude and rate of sprouting following an acute injury to the nervous system appear much greater in the immature brain. Recent work has revealed events at the cellular level that drive this regenerative process through activation of genes responsible for molecular growth-promoting programs.

A final anatomic mechanism involved in modifying neural connections in response to brain injury consists of a resting population of neural progenitor cells, which retain the capacity to proliferate, divide, and differentiate following injury, especially stroke, when activated by the correct signals. In addition, damage in the CNS also appears to initiate a cascade of molecular signals that recruit migrating neuroblasts into the areas of injury. Whether these cells, through neurogenesis, promote restoration of function in humans, however, has not been established.

Plasticity of the Nervous System

Another explanation for restoration of neurological function following injury is that the nervous system has developed characteristics that allow a certain degree of malleability both during development and in reaction to damage. Plasticity is a term that encompasses multiple capabilities of the nervous system to encode information in response to learning, as well as adapting to environmental changes. In the context of rehabilitation, plasticity may relate both to redundancy within the nervous system and to the process of vicarious functioning. Redundancy implies that there are latent neural connections and silent synapses, which can subserve a particular function if the primary control pathway is damaged. It is a compensatory strategy in which a damaged neural system subsequently comes to rely on new queues or different receptors, with resultant reorganization of the cortex. This type of acute adaptation has been well defined in experimental conditions. In human recovery, its role is gaining acceptance; the best evidence supporting its existence comes from fMRI and PET studies documenting recovery of function in young patients undergoing surgical hemispherectomy. Various neurologic functions, including motor performance and expressive language, can shift from a damaged area of brain to the corresponding location in the opposite hemisphere.

The process by which neural tissues not normally involved in performance of a particular task alter their characteristics to assume control of the task has been labeled vicarious functioning. Vicarious functioning most commonly occurs in an area of the brain adjacent to the injured site or systematically related to the damaged tissue. Evidence supporting this construct comes from experimental two-stage lesions, as well as PET studies involving the immature visual cortex. For example, in adults who lost sight at an early age, Braille reading not only activated the somatosensory cortex representing the reading fingers, but also the primary visual cortex. The concept of vicarious functioning implies a highly developed capability for CNS reorganization, which typically is not attributed to the mature nervous system. Thus, while the role of vicarious functioning in children is likely, its role for recovery in adults is less certain.

Mechanisms of Late Recovery

Recovery that occurs long past the onset of injury primarily is dependent upon the mechanism of functional substitution. This concept implies an overt or covert adaptation of an altered strategy in order to achieve a goal. It is a recovery of the "ends" and not a restoration of the "means to that end," in that the action performed is modified in order to fit the capabilities of undamaged nerve cells. The tissue subserving this recovery does not alter its intrinsic properties, but utilizes novel strategies to complete the task. An example of this is a paraplegic learning to propel a wheelchair with his upper extremities as a substitute for ambulating using the leg muscles. Since functional substitution is highly dependent upon new learning and repetitive problem-solving, neurorehabilitation can impact greatly on this type of recovery.

Clearly, recovery following damage to the nervous system is a highly complex and a remarkable series of processes. The postulated mechanisms appear to favor the immature or developing brain, thus accounting for the relatively better outcomes typically demonstrated in children. The proposed events of neural reorganization that emerge in response to injury are, for the most part, well-recognized, normal developmental processes of maturation, which are reactivated or potentiated in response to CNS damage. Hopefully, as our understanding of these mechanisms of recovery increases, there will come a time when neurorehabilitation therapy will be tailored to fit the particular circumstances of nervous system injury and restoration.

Principles of Pediatric Neurorehabilitation

Disorders involving the CNS represent a large proportion of all severe and complex disabilities, especially those secondary to trauma and other acquired injury. This situation is especially true in the pediatric population, where injury to or malformation of the brain and spinal cord accounts for the vast majority of children referred for rehabilitation. Pediatric neurologists therefore are uniquely positioned to contribute in a meaningful way to the discipline of pediatric rehabilitation.

Pediatric rehabilitation has several guiding principles based upon the nature of the discipline, as well as the age and developmental level of the patients requiring treatment. A fundamental principle of neurorehabilitation is that the process mandates a coordinated transdisciplinary team working in unison to provide integrated evaluations and therapeutic interventions. A variety of "nonmedical" issues, such as home and school accessibility, psychosocial adaptation to disability, and school reintegration, mandates that the team include individuals who can address these all-important considerations. A second essential principle is that the rehabilitation process must concentrate on strategies designed to effect true functional improvement, as opposed to enacting treatments that merely decrease symptoms without resulting in improvement in a patient's capabilities. In pediatric rehabilitation, this means establishing practical management decisions that are endorsed not only by the patient, but also by the family. In order to accomplish this goal, the team must have a clear understanding of the physical, emotional, cognitive, and social consequences of a child's injury.

The degree, extent, and rate of recovery, which varies significantly among children, as well as differences in functioning from setting to setting and task to task in a single child, mandate continual reassessment. As previously described, the immature brain's response to injury is both varied and dynamic. This evolving biologic recovery, in combination with substitute/alternative cognitive processes and movement patterns, necessitates an on-going program of assessment and reassessment. Additionally, progress from the baseline condition hopefully will be observed as a direct response to the therapeutic interventions. Rehabilitation, especially as it pertains to nervous system injury, has been described as a spiral management process in which, following an initial evaluation, a treatment program is initiated; this, in turn, is constantly revised and updated, based on successive reassessments, taking into consideration therapy-mediated improvements.

Another fundamental and distinguishing principle of pediatric rehabilitation is that these frequent reassessments of cognitive, motor, and psychosocial deficits, especially when resulting from acquired nervous system injury, must be guided by an understanding of normative development. Detailed understanding of the patterns of cognitive development during maturation is especially important in the rehabilitation of infants and children for several reasons. First, normative developmental milestones can be identified as sequential goals within an individual's therapy program. In addition, as a result of injury or illness, the pediatric patient typically loses age-appropriate developmental capabilities. As such, the manner in which therapy can be provided to the patient and the individual's ability to respond to it will be limited. This is most notable in children and adolescents early in the recovery process, who lack the developmental skills necessary to learn complex strategies upon which functional substitution is predicated. Finally, an understanding of cognitive development allows more accurate prediction of the long-term effects of cerebral injury sustained by young children. This is most pertinent for areas of brain subserving functions that normally mature later in childhood, such as executive functioning within the frontal lobes.

A final guiding principle of rehabilitation in the pediatric patient is that intervention should begin as soon as possible. Coma is not a contraindication to the initiation of rehabilitation management strategies, and thus, once the patient is medically stable, therapy can and should be instituted, even while the child is still in the intensive care unit. This early phase of intervention is designed to limit maladaptive behavioral habits and movement patterns, and to prevent or at least minimize complications that can take months to resolve, if not properly and promptly addressed following the acute injury. Specific goals include: prevention of physical deformities, such as contractures due to abnormal spasticity and prolonged immobilization; maintenance of skin integrity; and reduction in the manifestations of dysautonomia secondary to fluctuations in muscle tone or bladder distinction.

Medical Aspects of Acute Pediatric Rehabilitation Management

Nutritional support is a key element of the acute management process. In any child with an acquired nervous system injury, the risk for compromised nutrition is very high. There are a variety of causes that contribute to this risk, such as a hypermetabolic state resulting from systemic trauma and/or infection; delayed gastric emptying and intestinal dysmotility and stasis; oral pharyngeal dysfunction, which, even if recognized, can lead to aspiration pneumonia; and underestimation of caloric requirements necessary for repair and growth. Feeding through a nasogastric tube should be implemented while the patient is in the intensive care unit. An exception would be cases of major intra-abdominal injury; in these instances, hyperalimentation may be warranted. Oropharyngeal dysfunction and resultant swallowing difficulties secondary to bilateral cerebral hemisphere injury and/or lower cranial nerve involvement are an almost universal complication of acquired brain injury in the pediatric population. Thus, a detailed evaluation by a rehabilitation feeding team is mandatory. As neurological recovery proceeds, gradual introduction of oral feeding begins, with a commensurate decrease in supplemental alimentation based upon assessment of caloric need by a pediatric dietician.

Other medical issues often impact on acute neurorehabilitation management and, in addition, can impair the accuracy of on-going reassessment by the team of rehabilitation specialists. Fever and associated infection are a near-universal complication seen in pediatric patients with acute neurorehabilitation needs. In those with intracranial trauma, the possibility of CNS infection must be considered. In patients with penetrating cranial injury and basilar or compound skull fractures, the risk of bacterial meningitis and brain abscess is increased significantly. Sinusitis is a relatively common infection secondary to the frequent need for nasotracheal intubation or long-term na-sogastric tube utilization. Other equally obvious sources of infection include indwelling urinary catheters and intravascular lines. Fever of central origin secondary to hypo-thalamic injury also has been documented in children with acquired brain injury. The setting commonly is one in which other clinical features of dysautonomia are observed, most notably elevated heart rate and blood pressure. However, the diagnosis of fever of central origin is not a tenable one until all other sources of infection have been carefully evaluated and excluded, including drug-induced fever.

Dysautonomia, a syndrome characterized by simultaneous and paroxysmal sympathet-ic and muscle overactivity, typically follows severe traumatic, as well as other forms of acquired brain injury. The incidence varies between 5 and 12 percent in children, its presence correlating with the most severe injury and the worst prognosis. Auto-nomic changes include marked tachycardia, hyperventilation, hypertension, fever, and increased sweating; motor changes include (decerebrate or decorticate) posturing, dys-tonia, rigidity, and spasticity. Evidence-based treatment paradigms for dysautonomia in pediatric patients are nonexistent, with all evidence being anecdotal in nature. Ga-bapentin and bromocriptine have been reported to reduce the number and severity of paroxysms in pediatric patients, while in adults there is evidence that additional medications, such as propranolol, labetalol, clonidine, morphine, and midazolam, can be beneficial. Intrathecal baclofen also has been shown to be quite effective, even in children who are resistant to oral medications.

Disturbances in endocrine function, although less common than infection, also can complicate severe acquired brain injury. Damage to the pituitary and hypothalamic glands can produce the syndrome of inappropriate antidiuretic hormone secretion (SIADH), or conversely, central diabetes insipidus, in which ADH secretion is insuf-ficient. Although generally transient, both of these conditions mandate judicious fluid and electrolyte management, as well as pharmacologic treatment with desmopressin acetate in cases of diabetes insipidus.

Gastrointestinal disorders are also common in the pediatric population with acquired nervous system injury. These range from delayed gastric emptying and intestinal stasis to hemorrhage secondary to reflux esophogitis, gastric hyperacidity, and stress ulcers. Additionally, any child with a feeding tube is at risk for damage to the gastric muco-sa. Thus, prophylactic management with H_2 receptor blockers is indicated. Finally, in children with severe traumatic injuries involving the nervous system, there is a high incidence of skeletal fractures, typically of the long bones. Such fractures may not be apparent early on in the comatose patient or in children with spinal cord injury, but reveal themselves during the early course of neurorehabilitation treatment. Close co-ordination between the orthopedic surgeons and the therapy team in regard to range of motion exercises and weight-bearing status is essential to optimize the response to therapy.

Comprehensive Pediatric Rehabilitation Programs

Once the above noted medical and surgical issues have stabilized, a decision has to be rendered regarding the direction in which the rehabilitation process should proceed. In some children, recovery has been sufficiently rapid for discharge from the acute care setting and institution of outpatient therapy or a day treatment program to be appropriate. For others, progress has been and likely will continue to be very slow. In these cases, a subacute nursing center with less intense physiotherapy, occupational therapy, and speech therapy is a reasonable consideration. The final alternative of a dedicated pediatric rehabilitation program is indicated for the vast majority of children and adolescents with moderate to severe acute neurological injury. Typical management issues demonstrated by these patients include:

- Immobility – inability to walk, climb stairs, or transfer to/from a wheelchair.

- Dependence in self-care activities – drinking, eating, dressing, maintaining personal hygiene, and applying a brace or prosthesis.

- Aphasia with significant receptive or expressive dysfunction.

- Cognitive or perceptual motor dysfunction.

- Incontinence of bowel or bladder.

- Limited functional performance due to poorly controlled pain.

Another group recognized to benefit from an intensive inpatient program of rehabilitation therapy are those patients with severe neuromuscular deconditioning secondary to prolonged intubation and ventilatory support, with the concomitant need for pharmacological paralysis and sedation. This latter group includes many children who have received heart or lung transplants, even in the absence of any overt CNS injury.

Over the last several years, eligibility criteria for admission to comprehensive neurorehabilitation services have been developed and refined. At most major pediatric hospitals, these criteria include the following: a primary condition that is medically stable, but one that mandates intensive and multidisciplinary rehabilitation care; the premorbid physical and cognitive level of the child indicate potential for meaningful recovery; the patient is responsive to verbal or visual stimuli and has sufficient alertness to participate in the rehabilitation process; and the injury/illness diagnosis allows a reasonable expectation for improvement, with the potential to achieve clearly identifiable treatment goals within a reasonable period of time.

A comprehensive pediatric rehabilitation program should provide a very highly intensive service through a transdisciplinary coordinated team approach. Most programs mandate an initial minimum of 3 hours of therapy each day; as recovery proceeds and endurance improves, the duration and scope of treatment are expanded to a full day of activity. The program usually is supervised by a physician with specialized training and experience in one of the disciplines of rehabilitation medicine. Rehabilitation nursing care/supervision must be provided 24 hours a day. Although therapeutic interventions carried out by physical and occupational therapists and speech-language pathologists are the mainstay of any treatment program, most rehabilitation teams also include psychologists, social workers, child-life specialists, music therapists, chaplains, orthotists, and dieticians. In any program with a large number of children with acquired brain injury, a pediatric neuropsychologist is an essential member of the team. Our rehabilitation service also benefits from having horticultural and art therapists participate in the care of our patients. Formal written team evaluations typically occur at least every other week to assess progress and impediments to recovery; consider possible solutions to the impediments; reassess and adjust established goals; and develop and implement discharge plans.

Management of Spasticity

Almost every single patient requiring acute neurorehabilitation services will manifest alterations in tone as a result of injury or illness. In addition, spasticity is a characteristic feature of many chronic motor disorders affecting infants, children, and adolescents. In the pediatric population, spasticity is most commonly found in children with hypertonic forms of cerebral palsy. However, spasticity can result from any disorder causing damage to or abnormal development of nerve cells or pathways controlling motor movements, either in the brain or in the spinal cord. Thus, spasticity is commonly observed in children with brain tumors and those with vascular, traumatic, infectious, and hypoxic injury to the brain or spinal cord.

In the early phase following CNS injury, absent or reduced tone typically is encountered; over time, the pattern often evolves into spasticity as one part of the upper motor neuron syndrome. Spasticity is defined as an exaggerated response to passive movement of a limb, inducing a velocity-dependent involuntary resistance of the stretched muscle. Spasticity is characterized by excessive and inappropriately timed activation of skeletal muscles, which often interferes with a child's ability to move voluntarily in a normal fashion. The clinical manifestations of spasticity vary, depending upon the sites of injury within the CNS. Extent of damage, as well as intrinsic characteristics of recovery, influences the presentation of spasticity. However, in almost all pediatric patients, spasticity will impair passive movement and static postural alignment. In addition, impaired activation of voluntary movement, resulting in weakness and clumsiness, often may accompany spasticity. Spasticity must be differentiated from other manifestations of impaired movement, such as dystonia and rigidity, both of which typically occur within the context of an associated or a secondary injury due to ischemia and hypoxia.

Spasticity to any significant degree interferes with a child's control of voluntary movement, coordination, exercise tolerance, and range of motion in the joints. Invariably, this results in a state of excessive energy expenditure, compared to able-bodied children.

Spasticity typically impedes a child's independence in activities of daily living, and may cause pain and disturb sleep. In the more severely affected individuals, patient care often is especially difficult. Over time, spasticity reduces protein synthesis in muscles and impairs longitudinal growth; the end result typically is permanent shortening of muscles (contractures) and the development of bony deformities.

Treatment of spasticity should be predicated upon establishing goals that improve a child's functional capabilities. Thus, the number one reason for attempting to decrease spasticity in the pediatric population is to improve functional movement, either upper-extremity use in activities of daily living, or leg and trunk movement to achieve ambulation. Improvement of head, neck, and trunk posture by reducing spasticity may have additional benefits in some children: namely, better oral feeding and breath support for speech. It must be recognized, however, that spasticity may impart advantages in certain individual cases, including maintenance of muscle bulk and tone; support of circulatory function; assistance in transfers and ambulation; and assistance in activities of daily living. Once the goals of treatment have been established, decisions can be made as to which treatment option is most likely to achieve the desired success.

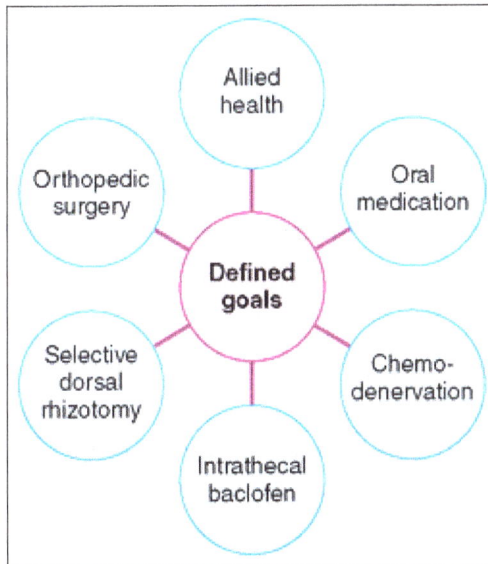

Treatment options for a child with spasticity.

Rehabilitation Therapy

The main focus of relieving spasticity in the earliest stages of rehabilitation is to minimize the complication of joint and muscle contractures, with a secondary goal of eliminating painful spasms. Management of spasticity in comatose or obtunded patients begins with proper positioning, range of motion exercises, and splinting, typically used in combination. Potential exacerbating factors, including external sensory stimuli (such as a catheter leg bag), irritation of the skin, bladder or bowel distention, and occult fractures, should be sought and eliminated. Range of motion (ROM) should be carried out daily to all joints, regardless of alteration of tone. As recovery ensues, the ROM exercises can be combined with physical treatment modalities and specific affected muscles targeted. Physical agents, such as heat, cold, water, and electrical stimulation, are effective adjuncts in the treatment of spasticity, with few side effects or contraindications. These measures likely reduce spasticity through inhibition and fatigue-induced direct relaxation of the spastic muscle. An alternative mode of action is via facilitation of the antagonists of a spastic muscle, creating relaxation by reciprocal inhibition. Finally, reduction in pain due to the use of physical modalities also may be operant in the reduction of tone. The degree of benefit varies among patients, but the duration of effect is rather short and time-dependent upon the length of the application.

Positioning is designed to facilitate proper postural alignment and symmetry and to correct weight-bearing distribution throughout the body as a means of minimizing flexible postural imbalances. Tone-inhibiting techniques of positioning can use gravity to stretch spastic muscles and thus promote relaxation. In the latter stages of recovery, proper position can facilitate active contraction of functionally weak muscle groups. Proper therapeutic alignment of the body is designed to counter the abnormal position assumed by the body at rest or when moved. Various reflex patterns (such as the asymmetric tonic neck reflex – ATNR), which may become activated depending on the location and extent of CNS damage, often underlie abnormal trunk and neck postures. Thus, specific positions or exercises that promote the disinhibited reflexes should be avoided. For example, supporting the head and neck properly will minimize the head-turning movements that typically elicit the ATNR and which, in turn, can further disrupt positioning of the remainder of the body.

Pediatric Physical Therapy

Pediatric physical therapy is concerned with the examination, evaluation, diagnosis, prognosis, and intervention of children, aged birth through adolescence, who are experiencing functional limitations or disability due to trauma, a disorder, or disease process.

Purpose

Pediatric physical therapy is indicated when a child has a pathology or suffers a trauma which results in an impairment leading to the loss of function and/or societal disability. Pathologies may include non-progressive neurological disorders such as cerebral palsy, which results from trauma to the brain during or shortly after birth. Children born with genetic syndromes, heart and/or lung defects, hydrocephalus, spina bifida, fetal alcohol syndrome, or drug addictionmay also be seen by physical therapists. Pathologies resulting in musculoskeletal impairments include, but are not limited to: juvenile rheumatoid arthritis, hemophilia, scoliosis, peripheral nerve injury, arthrogryposis, osteogenesis imperfecta, and muscular dystrophy. Acquired pathologies that may require physical therapy include traumatic brain injury, spinal cord injury, and cancer.

Pediatric physical therapists are employed in several different settings, including hospitals, outpatient clinics, and school systems. In the hospital, a pediatric physical therapist may work with patients such as those recovering from heart or lung conditions or surgery, burn trauma, orthopedic surgeries, or any number of other conditions. In addition, many neonatal intensive care units (NICUs) also employ physical therapists to evaluate and treat high-risk or premature infants . In an outpatient setting, the same children may be seen further along in their recovery. Children with lifelong conditions may be referred to outpatient clinics upon manifestation of secondary impairments. School physical therapists are employed to insure that children with disabilities or developmental difficulties are functioning adequately in their least restrictive environment.

In any case, the goal of treatment is to diminish impairments and functional limitations to prevent or decrease disability. Treatment may be focused on improving developmental tasks, motor planning, manipulation skills, balance, and/or coordination. The affected child may present with difficulties with ambulation, positioning, communication, attention, cognition, and/or motor function. All of these problems need to be addressed, as they can result in the inability to keep up with peers or perform work at school.

Precautions

Upon patient examination, a physical therapist collects the patient's history and does a systems study. The study includes assessment of the cardiovascular, respiratory, integumentary, musculoskeletal, and neuromuscular systems, including cognition. Physical therapists are educated in differential diagnosis for the purpose of identifying problems that are beyond the scope of physical therapy practice or require the attention of another health care professional.

Examination

Determining a child's need for physical therapy requires both qualitative and quantitative measures to gather information. Observation in natural settings, personal and family history, and subjective information from teachers or caregivers are all valuable pieces of the puzzle. A systems study should be performed, as discussed above. Through observation and measurement, active and passive range of motion and strength should be assessed. In addition, equilibrium and righting reactions and persistent abnormal reflexes should be noted. Posture and gait observation and assessment are essential for providing recommendations regarding exercises, seating, orthotics, and assistive devices.

Assessment of functional motor ability is often performed using a standardized test. In infants, tests often used include, but are not limited to: Movement Assessment of Infants, Peabody Developmental Motor Scales (PDMS), Test of Infant Motor Performance, Alberta Infant Motor Scale, and Bayley Scales of Infant Development II. Tests for children include the PDMS, Bruininks-Oseretsky Test of Motor Proficiency, and Gross Motor Function Measure. These tests look at the ability to perform tasks such as maintaining a prone position or rolling in infants, to walking a balance beam or throwing a ball in children.

Evaluation, Diagnosis and Prognosis

Although a child may have been given a medical diagnosis, the therapist should formulate a physical therapy diagnosis upon evaluation of the examination findings. The physical therapy diagnosis focuses not on the pathology (e.g., hydrocephalus), but rather on the dysfunctions toward which the therapist will direct intervention (e.g., decreased balance).

The prognosis encompasses a prediction of the level of function realistically attainable and the time period in which it will be accomplished. The prognosis includes the plan of care, which outlines treatment procedures and frequency, in addition to specifying long-term and short-term goals. In a rehabilitation or outpatient clinic setting, goal-setting may be more short-term than in an educational setting, where the tendency is to set yearly goals related to school function.

While goals often encompass the reduction of impairment to prevent functional limitations, reductions of primary impairment can help to prevent secondary impairment as well. For example, a goal focused on reduction of spasticity through proper positioning can help to prevent or diminish the occurrence of muscle shortening and joint contractures.

Intervention

Intervention involves the interaction between therapist and patient. It also includes communication with the family and other professionals as needed, including physicians, nurses, psychologists, occupational therapists, speech and language pathologists, physical therapist assistants, and social workers. In the educational setting, interactions also take place with classroom and physical education teachers, along with paraprofessionals.

Intervention encompasses the coordination and documentation of care, specific treatment procedures, and patient/family education. Physical therapists also must be skilled in recognizing the need to refer a patient back to a physician or recommend the services of other professionals as necessary. The physical therapist usually plays a key role in making recommendations or sometimes participating in the fabrication and fitting of orthoses, walking aids, and wheelchairs. In addition, the physical therapist is instrumental in choosing appropriate adaptive equipment, such as seating devices or standing frames, for the classroom or home.

Specific treatment procedures are numerous, falling into several categories: functional training for activities of daily living; therapeutic exercise; manual techniques such as mobilization and stretching; and therapeutic modalities. In 2001, evidence-based practice would require the use of recent motor control, motor development and motor learning theories as an umbrella over these treatment procedures. Motor control, development, and learning theories focus on the idea that several factors contribute to emergence of motor behavior. These factors include not only the central nervous system (CNS) as the driving force, but also biomechanical, psychological, social, and environmental components. Teaching and practice of skills under these theories is task-oriented and intermittent versus rote and repetitive. Higher-level learning takes place through problem-solving by the child rather than by the therapist's hands-on facilitation. Emphasis has also been placed on the importance of family-centered care, transdisciplinary service, and treatment in natural environments.

Treatment sessions may take place as frequently as once or twice a day in a rehabilitation setting, to once or twice a month in a school setting. Sessions may last 20 minutes to a full hour. Consultation with other professionals also takes place frequently during a patient's length of stay or a student's education.

Re-examination

A physical therapist is continually assessing a child's abilities and adjusting treatment appropriately. Some or all of the same tests and measures used during initial examination may be again used in order to evaluate progress and determine the need to modify, redirect or discontinue treatment.

Aftercare

Aftercare depends upon the setting in which the child has been treated. After a stay in a hospital, a child may be discharged with the recommendation to continue outpatient or school-based physical therapy. Upon discharge in any case, a physical therapist should provide recommendations for exercises or adaptations, if any, which should be continued at school or at home. In addition, a therapist may make suggestions regarding participation in programs such as adaptive sports leagues, therapeutic horseback riding, camps, etc.

Results

Although pediatric physical therapy addresses problems related to a wide variety of pathologies, the common goal usually is that functional activity increases and that disability decreases. In the case of non-progressive disorders, long-term retention of learned skills and the ability to transfer skills to different environments and situations are results of effective physical therapy intervention. In the case of progressive disorders such as muscular dystrophy, maintenance of capabilities and/or slowing of functional losses may be the goal.

Health Care Team Roles

The physical therapist and the physical therapist assistant, under the supervision of the physical therapist, are the direct providers of pediatric physical therapy. There are, however, many other key players. Although many states allow direct access to physical therapy, many require a referral from a physician. The physician usually provides the therapist with a prescription for physical therapy that outlines the medical diagnosis, and sometimes, precautions and recommendations. The child's physician and nurses also may provide valuable information regarding past medical history, surgical procedures, and medications.

Occupational therapists, speech and language pathologists, social workers, and psychologists also play important roles in the transdiciplinary provision of services. Physical therapists may work closely with these professionals to combine efforts toward fulfilling a child's maximum potential.

To summarize the various roles of a therapist in pediatric physical therapy, it is necessary to recognize, he or she is responsible for consultation, education, critical inquiry, administration, and supervision.

Consultation

There are many facets to the role of consultation. Physical therapists may be called upon to assist other health care professionals in determining whether or not physical therapy services are required for a specific patient, and which types of service are required. In addition, physical therapists may be asked to perform activities such as: assessing an environment or program for accessibility; providing opinions or recommendations on adaptations in the classroom, home or recreational arena; and making recommendations for compliance with the Individuals with Disabilities Education Act or the Americans with Disabilities Act.

Education

Physical therapists are responsible for educating patients and families, as discussed earlier. This education may include: general information about a disease and course of physical therapy treatment; teaching of home exercises and adaptations; instruction on prevention of secondary impairments; and suggestions for long-term wellness. In addition, pediatric physical therapists may be asked to provide information about disabilities to teachers or students in a school, or provide in-services to physical education teachers about adaptive sports. Pediatric physical therapists also are responsible for furthering their own education, mentoring future physical therapists and PT assistants, and increasing public awareness of areas in which physical therapists have expertise. The American Physical Therapy Association (APTA) offers a program for specialized certification, which is governed by the American Board of Physical Therapy Specialties (ABPTS) to facilitate the continuing education of physical therapists.

Critical Inquiry

Pediatric physical therapists have a responsibility to the profession to critically examine research findings and apply them when appropriate to their daily practice. In addition, physical therapists should look for ways to conduct and/or participate in research to evaluate the effectiveness of interventions and philosophies used in the profession.

Administration and Supervision

The pediatric physical therapist must be concerned with administrative activities related to human resources, equipment, finances, and facilities. Supervision of physical therapist assistants, student physical therapists and assistants, and physical therapy aides is often a responsibility. This responsibility may include monitoring quality of care and productivity as well.

References

- Neuromuscular-disorders, specialties-services-conditions: childrens.com, Retrieved 19 May, 2019

- Physiotherapy-Treatment-Approaches-for-Individuals-with-Cerebral-Palsy: physio-pedia.com, Retrieved 15 April, 2019

- Muscular-dystrophies, conditions-and-treatments-movement-disorders: childrensnational.org, Retrieved 19 June, 2019

- Pediatric-rehabilitation-methods-help, rehabilitation-medicine: acrm.org, Retrieved 18 April, 2019

- Pediatric-neurorehabilitation-medicine: clinicalgate.com, Retrieved 23 May, 2019

- Pediatric-physical-therapy, encyclopedias-almanacs-transcripts-and-maps: encyclopedia.com, Retrieved 16 July, 2019

Chapter 5

Role of Physical Medicine and Rehabilitation in Various Disorders

Physical medicine and rehabilitation has a wide domain which comprises of treatments for shoulder disorders, low back pain, knee injury, spinal cord injuries, Parkinson's disease, hemophilia, +-Guillain-Barre syndrome, etc. This chapter has been carefully written to provide an easy understanding of the aspects related to physical medicine and rehabilitation of various disorders.

Shoulder Disorders

Shoulder pain is a widespread problem and is responsible for a high percentage of patients presenting to general practice, causing absenteeism and labor complaints for sickness.

A lot of factors and conditions may contribute to shoulder pain. The most common cause is rotator cuff tendinopathy; its importance is linked not only to its high prevalence rate, but also because it is a disabling condition, causing high costs for health service.

As mentioned, rotator cuff injury is one of the most common shoulder disorders. Among these, the most common are tendinosis, partial thickness tear, and complete rupture. The incidence of the cuff injuries varies from 5 to 39%; it increases in the elderly population, being approximately 6 and 30%, respectively in patients aged below and above 60 years.

In this context, physical medicine and rehabilitation plays a fundamental role. The conservative approach consists of several interventions. The aim of these is to decrease shoulder pain and to regain shoulder function, with the goal to reduce the degree of impingement, decreasing swelling and inflammation, and minimizing the risk of further injuries. Many studies have shown that conservative therapy is the first-line treatment for shoulder disorders, in fact rehabilitative approach allows a reduction in pain feeling and symptoms within few weeks.

In literature, several studies have proposed conservative treatment for shoulder diseases, such as non-steroidal anti-inflammatory drugs (NSAIDs), cortisone injections, stretching and strengthening exercises, manual therapy, and physical energies (cryo-therapy, extracorporeal shock wave therapy (ESWT), laser therapy, ultrasounds, etc.) to reduce pain feeling and restore shoulder range of motion (ROM) and function.

Biomechanics

Understanding rotator cuff functions and shoulder biomechanics, it is crucial to understand shoulder disorders and their pathogenesis. The rotator cuff allows the stabilization of the glenohumeral joint, compressing the humeral head on the glenoid of the scapula. This mechanism is due to the equal and opposite action of the subscapularis anteriorly and infraspinatus and teres minor muscles posteriorly.

Scientific studies about shoulder biomechanics have explained precisely the contribution of every ligaments, tendons and muscles to shoulder stability. The action of rotator cuff is to compress the humeral head against scapular glenoid giving stabilization to the joint and allowing concentric rotation. Rotator cuff muscles play an important role in stabilizing glenohumeral joint through this compressive mechanism, in particular during mid-ranges motion in which ligaments are lax. Concavity compression mechanism is also important at end-ranges of motion, during which rotator cuff muscles protects ligaments by limiting the range of motion and decreasing strain, usually increased when shoulder reaches maximum abduction and extrarotation. When shoulder joint is in neutral position, rotator cuff muscles contribute equally in providing anterior stability. However, with glenohumeral joint in end-range abduction, subscapularis is a less effective stabilizer than other muscles, while the biceps brachii starts to play a role in joint stability.

The "concavity compression" is an important stability mechanism. The compression of the humeral head (convex), exercised by muscles of the rotator cuff, on the glenoid cavity (concave), maintains stable humeral epiphysis, in relation to translational forces. Resistance to joint subluxation is directly proportional to the depth of the articular concavity and to the compression force exerted by the muscles of the rotator cuff. Concavity compression, providing stability of glenohumeral joint, also depends on the extension of glenoid's articular surface (glenoid arc) available to accommodate humeral head.

Stabilization function is made evident when the disease is established; in fact, a rotator cuff tear results in the inefficiency of this mechanism with the consequent sliding of the humeral head upward. This is due to the action of the upper fibers of the deltoid muscle, resulting in a subacromial impingement.

The action of the rotator cuff muscles must be highly coordinated to be able to perform a specific movement. The muscles must work in coordination, as the rotation of the glen humeral joint does not have a fixed axis.

Tension loads acting on rotator cuff tendons can be divided into two types: concentric and eccentric. Concentric ones are generated when humerus has the same direction of cuff muscle, as it happens during abduction against resistance. These loads are better tolerated by the cuff insertion, which clears the acromion at low angles of elevation, protecting it from impingement by the coracoacromial arch. Eccentric tension loads are produced when the arm movement is opposed to the direction of cuff muscles direction. This occurs in example during active resistance to a downward force applied on the humerus. In fact, when the humeral head rotates with respect of the scapula, bending loads stress cuff tendons; cuff elasticity permits to resist these loads. Rotator cuff tendons are also subjected to compressive loads; an upwardly load presses the cuff between the humeral head and the coracoacromial arch. Furthermore, it has demonstrated a morphologic adaptation of the supraspinatus tendon with fibrocartilaginous areas in regions of compression, due to mechanical forces.

Every rotator cuff muscle origins on the scapula, which therefore influences the activity of these muscles. Therefore, rotator cuff performance is strictly related to the functional state of the scapula. When this bone is well stabilized, thus presenting the proper position in both static and dynamic tasks, it permits rotator cuff to work at an optimal level. However, alterations in scapular kinematics produce an unstable support to rotator cuff and consequently it affects the biomechanics of the shoulder. Scapular dysfunctions may be causative in rotator cuff disorders or may be the result of rotator cuff injuries, increasing the alteration.

Many authors have studied scapula kinematics in patients with rotator cuff diseases; alterations in scapular function have been found in most studies. In subjects with clinical symptoms or imaging demonstrating rotator cuff disorders, studies have demonstrated biomechanics alterations, especially scapular dyskinesia. Possible alterations are not consistent, with various combinations of changes like increase in upward rotation, decrease in posterior tilt and increase in internal rotation. However, the exact relationship between scapular dyskinesia and rotator cuff disorder is not completely clear; is dyskinesis a cause, an effect or a compensation.

Shoulder Disorders

Pathogenesis of rotator cuff injuries is not completely clear, but it may arise from extrinsic factors, impingement by structures surrounding the cuff, and intrinsic alterations of the tendon itself.

On the tendinous portion of the rotator cuff impingement by the coracoacromial ligament and the acromion itself is responsible for the characteristic "impingement syndrome". A peculiar proliferative spur and ridge on the anterior lip and undersurface of the acromial anterior process has been found; furthermore, in many studies this area has shown erosions.

Anatomical changes may excessively narrow the subacromial space, in which rotator cuff tendons pass through, and include acromial shape variations (i.e. hooked acromion), orientation of the acromial angle or prominent osseous changes of the inferior portion of the acromion-clavicular joint. In 1986, Bigliani described the important role of acromion shape, as an extrinsic mechanism, in rotator cuff tendinopathy; acromion classified into three types based on different shapes: Flat (Type I), Curved (Type II) and Hooked (Type III).

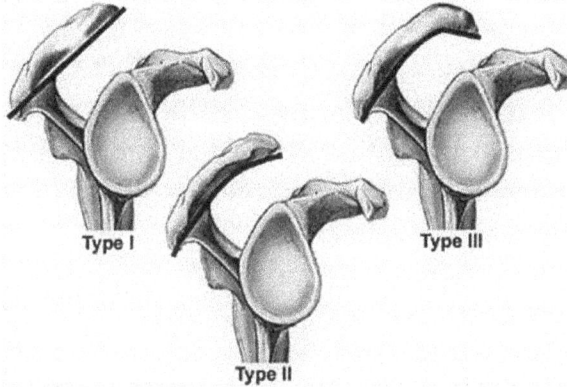

Type I

Type III

Type II

Bigliani classification for acromial in different shapes.

Association between acromion shape and severity of rotator cuff disorder has been well documented, with a greater prevalence of hooked acromion in subjects with subacromial impingement syndrome and full thickness tears. Alterations of shoulder kinematics, postural abnormalities, rotator cuff muscles deficits and decreased extensibility of pectoralis minor are biomechanical factors which can lead to rotator cuff tendons compression. In addition, shoulder kinematic alterations can cause a dynamic reduction of the subacromial space (compressing rotator cuff tendons) due to a superior shift of the humeral head or an altered scapula biomechanics that leads acromion sliding downwards.

Recent studies suggested that subacromial bursa is a pro-inflammatory membrane responsible for shoulder pain and other subacromial disorders. Blaine demonstrated that inflammatory cytokines, such as Tumor necrosis factor (TNF), Interleukin 1 (IL-1), Interleukin 6 (IL-6), cyclooxygenase-1 (COX-1) and cyclooxygenase-2 (COX-2), increase in subacromial bursal in subjects suffering from bursitis and rotator cuff syndrome. It should also be pointed out that IL-1 and IL-6 play an important role as mediators of collagen catabolism.

Peritendinous alterations in rotator cuff disorders are thought to be a secondary phenomenon. Chandler showed that the increased tension in the coracoacromial ligament, due to tendinopathy, stimulates the neoformation of bone on the underside of the acromion, which may result in an impingement syndrome leading to enthesopathy.

Acromial lateral sloping or glenoid version is structural features which play an important role in rotator cuff pathology as extrinsic factors. As mentioned in the previous paragraph, acromion shape influences supraspinatus tendon as it passes under the coracoacromial arch. Even a forward scapula posture, caused by forward head posture and increased kyphosis in combination, can reduce the subacromial space.

Intrinsic factors, causing rotator cuff tendinopathy, affect tendon morphology and performance. There is growing evidence in literature supporting the fundamental role of these mechanisms in shoulder disorders.

Intrinsic mechanisms, such as aging processes, poor vascularity and altered biology, lead to tendon degradation also influencing tensile forces and altering loads.

A reduction in vascular supply of tendons is implicated in rotator cuff tears pathogenesis. In 1934, Codman described for the first time the "critical zone" (1 cm area between the insertion of supraspinatus tendon at greater tubercle and myotendinous junction) which represents the most common site for tendon injury due to its reduced vascularity.

Tendon degeneration is the expression of an increased production by tenocytes of metalloproteinase enzymes (MMP); this means that tendon tears are an active and cell-mediated process. The hypothesis is that rotator cuff tears are the results of an imbalance between tendon synthesis and degradation, maybe due to the failed regulation of MMP activity in response of repeated mechanical strains. Tendon degeneration is further evident as it has demonstrated an increase in sulfated glycosaminoglycans (GAG) in supraspinatus tendinosis. Sulfated GAG are associated with acute inflammation and new matrix formation, as well as amyloid production. A demonstrated that supraspinatus chronic tears were characterized by 70% amyloid deposition on tendon context, unlike only 25% in patients suffering from acute traumatic injuries.

Another feature that may lead to shoulder disorders is genetics; it seems to be related to the polymorphism of genes which regulates collagen synthesis, like the one found in Achilles tendinopathy. However, this is just a hypothesis since no genes were identified till now as risk factors for rotator cuff diseases.

Other factors can influence mechanical properties and tensile loads response including tendon geometry, due to collagen fiber alignment. Among tendon alterations, it is important to highlight tendon irregularity and thinning, observed in subjects suffering from degenerative rotator cuff tendinopathy; these conditions influence mechanical properties. Even aging has been observed to be a negative factor for tendon degeneration. Biomechanical studies showed a reduced elasticity and a decreased tensile strength in tendons with aging. Histological studies about rotator cuff tendons showed degenerative changes (calcifications and fibrovascular proliferation) in elderly in comparison to young people, both groups without history of shoulder disorders. Furthermore, aging causes a reduction in total sulfated GAG and proteoglycans in supraspinatus tendon.

Other scientific researches demonstrated in elderly people a reduction of type I collagen and an increase in type III, weaker and more irregularly; however there is no consensus in literature whether these changes are related with aging or a secondary consequence of healing processes to repeated microtrauma (or overuse).

An interesting classification is the one developed by Celli that divides the old denomination "shoulder periarthritis" in four clinical presentations, depending on the type, localization and pain:

- Acute anterior shoulder: Where inflammation is limited to the supraspinatus tendon and/or to the long head of the biceps tendon.

- Global acute shoulder: Pain is acute and inflammation compromised subdeltoid bursa.

- Chronic anterior shoulder: Pain is chronic and localized on the anterior region.

- Global chronic shoulder: Even in this case the pain is chronic, but it affects the whole shoulder.

This classification has the advantage of easy application, but there is no immediate correlation with the cause of degeneration. The most common cause of shoulder pain is an inflammation of the bursae around the glenohumeral joint. The most affected is the subacromial bursa, located between the acromion and the tendons of rotator cuff, but also subdeltoid, subscapularis and subcoracoid bursae may be affected.

Pain is localized on the side of the proximal part of the arm, but it may also extend distally if the inflammatory process involves subdeltoid bursa, which often communicates with the subacromial one. Movements accentuate symptoms, particularly active abduction, that is markedly limited by pain.

Rotator Cuff Tendinosis

The incidence of rotator cuff tendinopathy and degenerative tears increases in aging and it is 40% in subjects over 70 years of age.

Rotator cuff tendinosis is due to disorganization in collagen fibers morphology and to alterations in tendon ultrastructure. Earlier studies showed histopathological changes associated with rotator cuff tendinosis: tendon fibers thinning and consequently ultrastructural alterations, cellular apoptosis, granulation tissue production and fibro-cartilaginous changes. The risk of progression, which can lead to full tendon rupture, is related to these histopathological changes.

Hyaline and myxoid degeneration, which can affect collagen fibers, already occur in the degenerated tendon. The consequence of this is a reduction in tensile resistance that predisposes the tendon to rupture.

In degenerated tendon, healing processes are altered. In fact, the standard composition and structure of the osteotendinous insertion site, with the transition from non-mineralized to mineralized fibrocartilage, is not achieved. The causes of this poor healing process are multifactorial, but correlated to an inadequate and disorganized expression of the cytokines responsible for the formation of the complex structure and composition of the enthesis.

Other factors that may influence healing processes are the presence of inflammatory cells in the osteotendinous insertion site and a small number of stem cells in the tendon-bone interface, which hamper physiological scar formation.

Healing process occurs in three steps:

- Inflammatory phase.

- Repairing phase.

- Remodeling phase.

An alteration during one of these phases leads to a bad regenerative process. Recent studies demonstrated the importance of the inflammatory phase, during which there is an increase of neutrophils, macrophages and mast cells in rotator cuff lesions in animal and human models. Millar evaluated rotator cuff tendon samples taken by biopsy during repairing phase. They observed significant infiltration of mast cells and macrophages in earlier phase of tendinopathy. Subsequently macrophages produce transforming growth factor-$\beta1$ (TGF-$\beta1$), which stimulates collagen formation and proteinase activity.

Fibrovascular scar is probably produced during this phase thanks to the action of macrophages. During the repairing phase of healing process, fibroblasts activation determines the expression of various cytokines, such as basic fibroblast growth factor (bFGF), insulin-like growth factor (IGF-1), platelet-derived growth factor-b (PDGF-b), vascular endothelial growth factor (VEGF), bone morphogenic protein-12 (BMP-12), BMP-13 and BMP-14.

Calcific Tendonitis

Calcific tendonitis can be potentially included in the sum of rotator cuff diseases. Its prevalence is estimated between 2.7 and 20% according to radiographies of asymptomatic adults. Usually occurs between the age of 40 and 50, with a higher prevalence in female sex and in sedentary workers. The probability of becoming symptomatic, both acute and chronic, has been estimated to be higher than 50%.

A Maugars pointed out that between 7 and 17% of patients suffering from chronic shoulder pain was due to tendon calcification.

Calcific tendonitis is not simply a degenerative disorder, since calcification is not histologically associated with necrosis or tissue damage, but it is a cell-mediated process similar to an incomplete endochondral ossification.

One of the first authors to describe the calcium deposits cycle was Uhthoff who divided it into two phases: a formative and resorptive one. Other authors subdivided the cycle into three phases: pre-calcification (asymptomatic), calcification (impingement) and post-calcification (acute).

A more complete classification divided this cycle into four phases: pre-calcific phase, during which the fibrocartilaginous transformation occurs in the tendon context in a completely asymptomatic manner; formation phase that consists of the deposition of hydroxyapatite crystals within the tendon; re-absorbing phase, characterized by the release of these crystals and finally post calcific recovering phase.

It is therefore evident that there is currently no standardized histological classification for tendon calcifications in literature.

In concern to the radiographic aspects of calcification, many studies converge on Gartner's classification, whereby three kinds of deposits can be identified. Type I refers to a well-defined and dense deposit, type II identifies a well-distinguished but radiotransparent deposit and finally, type III has a radiotransparent structure but with marginal margins.

In fact, the classification of the French Arthroscopic Society also identifies three types of calcifications, indicating them with letters A, B and C, which reproduce the description of Gartner.

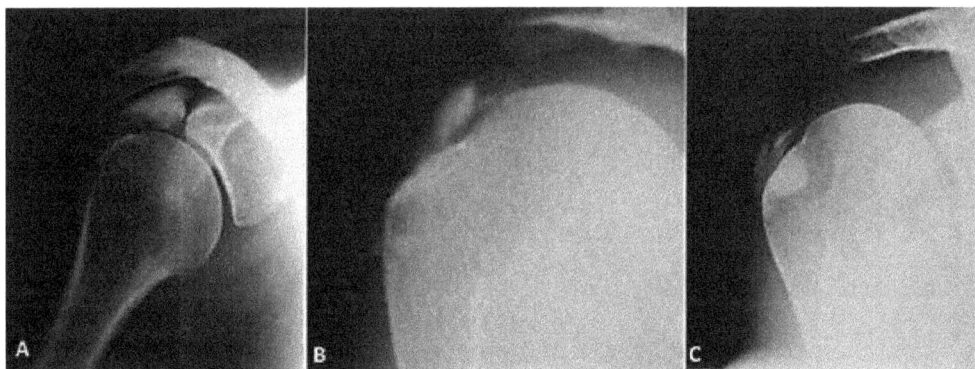

Classification of calcifications by French Arthroscopic Society. A: Dense deposit and well-defined margins, C: nubecular deposit, margins not defined. B: intermediate between the two previous types.

The fundamental concept is that radiographic classification is not sufficient on its own, but correlation with the clinical data is always necessary.

Subacromial Bursitis and Impingement

The subacromial bursa is the largest and most complicated bursa in human body. In a 1934 book, Codman affirmed that it behaves as a secondary scapula-humeral joint, although it is not composed of cartilage tissue. Therefore, he highlighted the functional issue of subacromial bursa. In 1972, Neer further emphasized this point of view in his studies on impingement syndrome. Moreover, in other studies, he suggested that subacromial bursa is an inflammatory membrane that can lead to pain through nociceptors endings stimulation. Santavirta found a majority of CD-2 and CD-11b mononuclear cells in the bursa of patients suffering from subacromial bursitis. Yanagisawa also demonstrated an increased expression of VEGF in patients with impingement syndrome, thus pointing out chronic inflammation and increased vascularity. Other studies demonstrated the increased expression of pain mediators (substance P) in the subacromial space in subjects with impingement syndrome.

Despite these evidences about subacromial bursa, the changes in biochemical mediators expression, implicated in subacromial impingement syndrome pathogenesis, have not yet completely identified. These investigations were carried on to determine the role of subacromial bursa in impingement syndrome; the question is if the bursa behaves as a pathological or a reparative tissue.

During bursitis, there is a reduction of the overall subacromial space, which may lead to an increased compression of tissues inside. During subacromial impingement syndrome, it has been demonstrated tendons degeneration, due to inflammatory processes or tension overload in shoulder mobilization (e.g. during work activities).

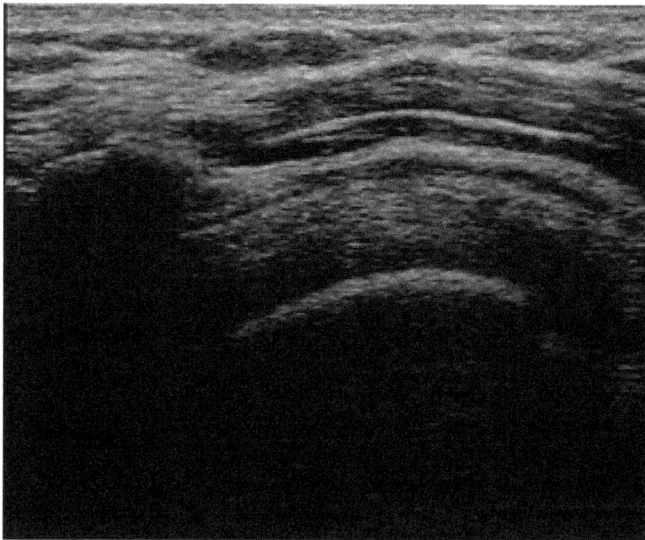

Subacromial bursitis: ultrasound imaging.

Impingement syndrome classification was first developed by Neer in 1983 and it is based on histopatological damage of tissues. He defined this syndrome as a mechanical-compressive lesion of tissues of the subacromial space and he identified three progressive stages: first stage ("edema and hemorrhage stage") is typical in patients aged 25 or less with a history of overhead use of the upper limb during sport or work; second stage is defined by further deterioration of rotator cuff tendons and subacromial bursa, and it usually affects 25–40 years old patients; last stage, the third one, is characterized by bone spurs and partial or full-thickness tendon rupture affecting subjects aged 40 or more.

Rotator Cuff Tears

Rotator cuff tears represent approximately one-third of medical visits for shoulder pain, but sometimes it is a problem difficult to diagnose. Among patients suffering from shoulder pain, rotator cuff tears are the most common cause, especially in subjects aged 60 or more. The incidence of this pathology increases with age; moreover, studies on cadavers have noticed 30% of cases with rotator cuff tears. As mentioned, literature agrees that the incidence increases with age. Yamamoto et al. observed a prevalence of full-thickness tears of 20.7% in a sample population, mean age 57.9 years, with or without symptoms. In a 2006 autopsy studies, evaluating 2553 shoulders (mean age 70.1 years), it observed a prevalence of 18.5% for partial-thickness tears and 11.8% for full lesions. Rotator cuff tears are very common, so the pathological history and the clinical examination play a critical role, especially in subclinical cases.

Pathogenesis of rotator cuff tears is complex and multifactorial. For this reason, there are two different schools of thought, according to which tendon injuries can be due to intrinsic or extrinsic factors. Codman had already described the intrinsic theory according to which tendon degenerates in the critical area of hypovascularity; this area is 1 cm from the insertion of supraspinatus to the humeral head. Besides this, due to its low vascularization, it is also an area with low healing capacity. According to extrinsic theory, the cuff tendons, flowing into the subacromial space (i.e. between the acromion, the coracoacromial ligament and the humeral head) can be compressed and then injured.

The majority of rotator cuff tears affected supraspinatus and infraspinatus tendons; these are described as postero-superior cuff tears. On the contrary, antero-superior tears are less common and typically extend anteriorly involving rotator interval or subscapularis tendon. Partial tears consist of a partial disruption of tendon fibers without communication among bursal and articular spaces.

The average normal thickness of rotator cuff tendons is between 8 and 12 mm. The depth of tear defines the degree of lesion. Codman classified tendon tears in three types:

- Bursal-side tear (BT) confined to the bursal surface of the tendon.

- Intratendinous tear (IT), which is localized within tendon thickness.

- Joint-side tear (JT) located on the joint side of the tendon.

Another classification proposed by Neer divided the condition of pain, inflammation, oedema and hemorrhage as stage I, tendinous fibrosis as stage II and fibers rupture as stage III.

Taking into account the average thickness of supraspinatus tendon, Ellman classified rotator cuff tears: grade I consists of a tear depth lower than 3 mm (or involving less than 25% of tendon thickness); grade II characterized by a depth between 3 and 6 mm or 50% of thickness; grade III involves more than 6 mm or more than 50% of thickness. In full-thickness tears a complete fibers disruption brungs to a direct communication between subacromial and glenohumeral spaces.

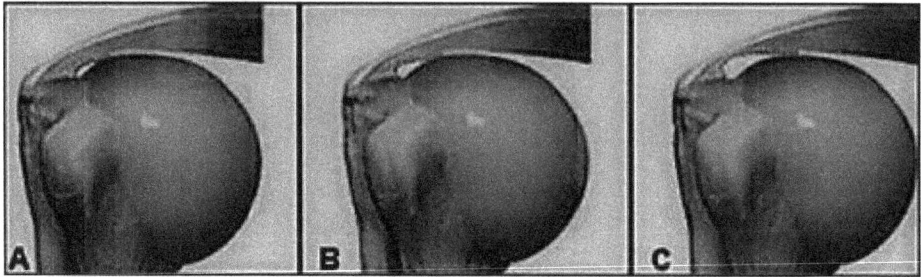

Ellman classification of rotator cuff tears. A: grade I; B: grade II; C: grade III.

Tables: Further classifications of rotator cuff tears are shown in tables.

Small	<1 cm
Medium	1–3 cm
Large	3–5 cm
Massive	>5 cm

Table: Cofield classification (by tear size).

Stage 1	Proximal stump lies close to its bony insertion.
Stage 2	Proximal stump retracted at level of humeral head.
Stage 3	Proximal stump retracted at glenoid level.

Table: Patte classification (by cuff tears retraction).

Stage	Muscle description
0	Completely normal muscle.
I	Some fatty streaks.
II	Amount of muscle is greater than fatty infiltration.
III	Amount of muscle is equal to fatty infiltration.
IV	Amount of fatty infiltration is greater than muscle.

The greater the size of the lesion, the extent of retraction and the quantity of fatty muscle atrophy, the less the chance of healing from rotator cuff tear. The natural history of the lesion is the further increase in size over time. Therefore, for example, partial thickness tears become total lesions and, referring to Cofield's classification, small-sized tears tend to evolve toward massive lesions.

Frozen Shoulder

Frozen shoulder, or adhesive capsulitis, is a painful and disabling condition of unknown etiology caused by a spontaneous contracture of the glenohumeral joint in absence of an evident previous event, resulting in reduction of joint motion. This debilitating condition affects from 2 to 5% of the general population and its prevalence increases to 10–38% in patients with comorbidities, such as hypothyroidism, diabetes, increased body mass index and cervical spondylosis. This condition is more common in women and in non-dominant shoulders. The mean age of onset is 50–55 years.

The currently recognized classification identifies as a primary frozen shoulder a condition with any clearly identifiable etiopathogenetic cause, and as secondary a condition triggered by a well-defined cause. The last one, is further subdivided into intrinsic, extrinsic and systemic.

Table: Frozen shoulder classification.

Primary adhesive capsulitis	Secondary adhesive capsulitis		
Idiopathic (of unknown etiology or condition)	Systematic • Thyroid disease • Hyperlipidemia • Hypoadrenalism • Chronic obstructive pulmonary disease (COPD) • Osteopenia/reduced bone mineral density • Duputreyn's disease • Ischemic heart conditions • Diabetes mellitus	• Extrinsic • Cardiac or breast surgery • Cerebrovascular accident • Cervical radiculopathy	Intrinsic Impingement Tendinopaty Osteoarthrits Dislocation or shoulder trauma

Neviaser describe this state as *adhesive capsulitis* to emphasize the inflammatory component affecting the capsule, multiregional areas of synovitis and synovial angiogenesis. Histological findings attribute to neoangiogenesis the growth of new nerves in the capsuloligamentous complex of these patients and this may be the explanation of the pain associated with capsulitis.

Immunocytochemical analysis on arthroscope biopsy material revealed the presence of chronic inflammatory cells predominantly made up of mast cells, T cells, B cells and macrophages, as well as the presence of fibrosis that results from mast cell infiltrate, which typically regulate the proliferation of fibroblasts.

Frozen shoulder seems to be the result of failure of the healing process after an initial inflammatory phase, characterized by an excess of cytokines and growth factors with fibroblasts accumulation that in part differentiate into myofibroblasts. They exert tractions on new collagen deposits with stiffening of the capsule.

The diagnosis is essentially clinical, based on the evidence of the reduction of the ROM (range of motion) in particular in extrarotation, elevation and intrarotation of the glenohumeral joint, in the absence of X-ray lesions. This is accompanied by pain at the insertion of the deltoid and muscular weakness. Radiographic images are not helpful, unless in the case of associated pathologies, such as fractures, arthritis and metallic implants. In selected cases, with suspected association with rotator cuff tendinopathy or impingement syndrome, we can refer to magnetic resonance imaging.

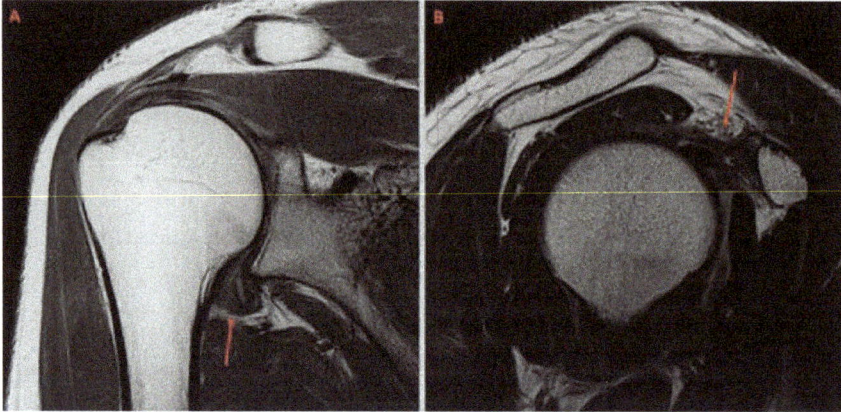

Frozen shoulder at MRI. Coronal PD (A): thickening of the axillary recess of the glenohumeral joint; sagittal PD (B): inflammation in the rotator cuff interval.

The clinical presentation is indicative of the stage of the adhesive capsulitis:

- Preadventive stage: Patients have mild pain at the end of the range of motion and this condition is often mistakenly diagnosed as impingement syndrome.

- "Freezing" stage: Is often characterized by a high level of discomfort and a high level of pain and a progressive loss of ROM.

- "Frozen" stage: Is characterized by significant stiffness, but less pain.

- "Thawing" stage: In this phase we have painless stiffness and motion that typically improves by remodeling.

Clinical Presentation

The diagnosis is based essentially on clinical examination, exclusion of other pathologies and normal glenohumeral radiographs. Initial evaluation of global postural assessment should be perform before focusing on the shoulder, because shoulder pain is often associated with thoracic and cervical spine alignment that alters the scapula's rest position. Postural abnormalities related to shoulder pain, include extension of the atlanto-occipital joints, reduction of physiological cervical lordosis, increase of dorsal kyphosis, protrusion (abduction) of the scapula with rotation downward and internal rotation of the humerus. All these results in neuro-musculoskeletal changes.

A thorough collection of the patient's medical history is used to detect if pain origins really from shoulder whether it is a referred pain from other anatomical structures. It is frequently reported that the pain in the shoulder is actually coming from the cervical spine, in which case the irradiation along the upper limb pain, radicular pathology reaches generally until the hand and the fingers, while the pain that starts from the shoulder radiates up and not past the elbow.

The shoulder physical examination can be expressed in the following steps: inspection, palpation, mobility and specific functional tests. The inspection is usually negative, while palpation may aid in the diagnosis. Palpation should include all the articulation of the scapular girdle and all the rotator cuff muscles trying to overcome with appropriate maneuvres the deltoid that covers a large part of the rotator cuff. During the palpation, must be taken simultaneously consider several aspects. They are: the tenderness, the swelling, changes in temperature, the deformity, both obvious and hidden, the muscle characteristics and the relations between the various structures. The motion of both shoulders should be assessed actively and passively. Forward elevation and elevation in the scapular plane as well as internal and external rotation with the arm at the side and in 90° of abduction should be performed.

Tests of affected muscles against resistance are imperative to formulate a correct diagnosis.

Neer test: The doctor is placed behind the patient, with one hand passively he raises his arm in internal rotation and abduction, while with the other stabilizes the scapula. If the patient refers pain in an arc of movement between 70° and 120°, the test shows a conflict between the greater tuberosity and the humeral the acromion.

Hawkins test: It is performed with arm at 90° of flexion front and elbow flexed to 90°; in this position the physician, in front of the patient and imprints an internal rotational movement of the glenohumeral joint. Pain located below the acromioclavicular joint with internal rotation is considered a positive test result and it is indicative of inflammation of the subacromial bursa or of an impingement of all structures that are located between the greater tubercle of the humerus and the coracohumeral ligament.

Palm-up test: The examiner contrasts the movement of the patient to elevate the arm with the elbow in extension and palm of the hand facing up. If the test shows pain is positive to a lesion of the long head of the humeral biceps.

Jobe test: The examiner stands in front of the patient keeps his arms positioned at 90° of abduction, 30° of anterior flexion and maximum intra-rotation (thumbs pointing to the ground). The examiner lowers arms against the patient's resistance against exerting a downward thrust. The test is positive for the supraspinatus muscle if the affected limb is lowered, regardless of whether or not the presence of pain.

Other tests can be used, such as Yocum test, the horizontal adduction test, the painful arc sign, the empty can test, the drop arm test, the Speed test, the Yergason test and the Pattes test.

Clinical evaluation can completed with assessment scales like Constant-Murley scale or simple shoulder test (SST).

The Constant-Murley score is an ordinal scale used in all pathologies of shoulder (not only for the instability), with a score ranging from 0 to 100 (100 = normal shoulder). The scale investigates four areas through the pain (15 points), activities of daily living (20 points), strength (25 points) and the range of motion (40 points). In this way it achieved a full assessment of the level of pain and disability related to the activities of daily living.

The "simple shoulder test" (SST) is a binary scale used for all shoulder pathologies that involves the administration of 12 questions to the patient (normal score = 12). The questions are used to assess the perceived pain and the ability to perform certain activities of daily living. The DASH is halfway between a generic test (as the Short Form) and a specific test for the shoulder, it can use to complete the assessment.

Imaging studies are commonly used to identify and differentiate the source of the injury.

Conservative Approach

The conservative approach avails of different kind of treatments, whose main purpose is to reduce pain and other signs of inflammation, recover function and prevent further joint damage.

A great number of studies support the conservative approach as the main treatment for the mildest forms of shoulder pain due to adhesive capsulitis. The natural course of the frozen shoulder leads to healing in more or less long times. To reduce pain faster and recover the articular functionality, we can intervene with several alone or combinated therapies, such as physical therapy (ultrasound, lasers, hyperthermia, electro-analgesia and shock waves), intra-articular corticosteroid injection, intra-articular saline hydrodilation with distention and eventual rupture of the glenohumeral joint capsule, intra-articular sodium hyaluronate injection into the glenohumeral joint, suprascapular nerve block, shoulder manipulation under anesthesia, oral corticosteroid or NSAIDs (non-steroidal anti-inflammatory drugs) and analgesics. In case of failure of these therapies, the alternative is to proceed with open or arthroscopic synovectomy and glenohumeral capsular releases.

Extracorporeal Shock Wave Therapy

Since 1980, the extracorporeal impact waves have been used in different conditions, initially to destroy kidney stones. Investigating the side effects on the surrounding tissues, it was understood that they could also find use in the treatment of musculoskeletal disorders. The effect on these tissues is dose-dependent: high doses tend to have destructive effects, low doses have regenerative effects.

The recommended energy limit should be beneath 0.28 mJ/mmq, above which necrotic effects prevail; ESWT is performed without anesthesia, even on larger areas; their application also on open growth plates seems to be safe.

The regenerative effect of ESWT is the consequence of the activation of gene expression for growth factors or cytokines and fibroblast proliferation. Mechanical stimulation is converted by tendon tissue in enhancement of TGF-β1 gene expression and increase of collagen I and collagen III.

The phenomenon of mechanosensing is particularly clear in bone tissue, due to its structure and physiology: it acts like a piezoelectric. After ESWT exposure, bone shows: osteogenic differentiation of mesenchymal stem cells expression of nitric oxide synthase (eNOS), vascular endothelial growth factor (VEGF) that lead to neoangiogenesis and accelerate tissue regeneration and healing bone regeneration, starting from periosteum stimulation direct stimulation of osteoblasts and indirect reduction of osteoclasts activity.

In addition, the increase in NOS appears to be involved in another signaling pathway leading to the reduction of pro-inflammatory factors. It has been seen that NOS exerts an inhibitory action on nuclear factor kappa-light-chain-enhancer of activated B cells (NF-κB), hence the role in production of proinflammatory cytokine and leukocytes recruitment, generating pain and phlogosis, are blocked.

Other mechanism is the production of NO and VEGF resulting in neoangiogenesis that improves blood supply promoting tissue repairing and wash-out of algogenic and noxious substances.

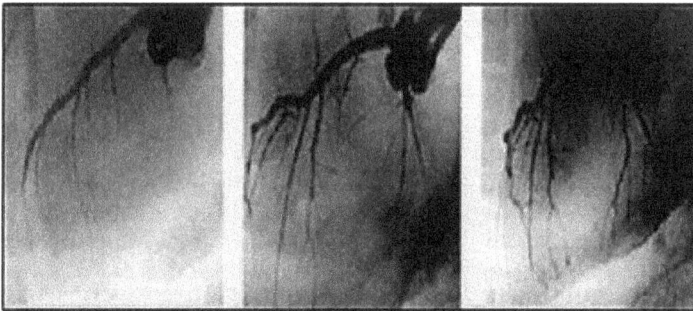

Coronary neovascularization after 4 weeks of shock wave therapy.

ESWT intervene in pain modulation also by release of endogenous analgesic sustances P and calcitonine gene-related peptide (CGRP) and according to the gate control. About the gate control, Saggini, claim that a hyperstimulation-like shock waves, activate the descending inhibitory system, blocking following nociceptive stimuli in the posterior column of the spinal cord. In addition, ESWT modify substances P and CGRP levels, damaging peripheral small unmyelinated fibers, responsible of immediate release of the algogenic peptide. All these mechanisms make ESWT suitable to treat various musculoskeletal disorders, such as calcific tendonitis, epicondylitis, osteoarthritis and long bone fracture.

ESWT has proved to be a valid option in the treatment of calcifying tendinitis of the shoulder. A study based on a meta-analysis showed the power of ESWT to intervene in case of calcific tendinitis, promoting resorption of the calcifications using high energy density (conventional limit set at 0.20 mJ/mmq, less than this intensity was labeled low-energy). Functional outcome (Constant-Murley score) and radiographic resorption (chance of complete resorption) of the deposits after 3 months, showed that high-energy ESWT is more effective than low-energy ESWT. The effect on calcifications is not merely mechanical as in the case of kidney stones, but rather biochemical induces interstitial and extracellular changes, enhancing tissue regeneration.

Few studies specifically address the application of ESWT in frozen shoulder. One of the study, recruited 36 patients divided into 2 groups: one received shock waves (1200 shocks with energy between 0.1 and 0.3 mJ/mmq) and one sham. Pain and disability score were assessed with the Shoulder Pain and Disability Index (SPADI) questionnaire before and after the therapy, and 2 and 5 months after the treatment. The results show a positive effect on recovery of frozen shoulder that was faster than sham group.

Another research compare ESWT (1000 shock waves, with energy between 0.01 and 0.16 mJ/mmq) with conservative physical therapy, both group treated twice a week for six weeks. Pain and function were assessed, respectively, with visual analogue scale (VAS) and patient-specific functional scales (PSFS). Both group showed significant decreases in VAS and PSFS, the ESWT group reported lower score then the control group.

ESWT is therefore a possible way to treat the frozen shoulder, especially if we consider the fact that it is a safe, non-invasive and low cost procedure.

Intra-articular Injections

Intra-articular drug administration offers several advantages: increased bioavailability, reduced systemic effects and fewer side effects. Moreover, most joints can be accessed accurately, especially under ultrasound guidance.

Intra-articular injections into the glenohumeral joint are commonly performed to treat different conditions affecting this articulation, such as osteoarthritis, adhesive capsulitis and rheumatoid arthritis. Despite the widespread use of this treatment, there are no standard criteria for their performance.

With regard to this type of therapy applied to the treatment of shoulder pain, two substances are used: corticosteroids and hyaluronic acid. The pharmacological properties of corticosteroids are well known, in accordance with them, this procedure is recommended in the acute phase. The risks associated with corticosteroid injection are limited if performed by experienced hands and in patients eligible for such procedure. Injection should be avoided in patients with septic arthritis, bacteremia and in immunocompromised patients.

The main purpose in treating the frozen shoulder is to reduce the loss of function and to give relief to pain that significantly limits movement. In the case of adhesive capsulitis, intra-articular administration of corticosteroids is generally associated with conventional physical therapy. A systematic study of 25 studies from 1947 to present, compares infiltrations with manipulation under anesthesia, physical therapy and distension of the joint capsule. In all cases it is clear that intra-articular administration of corticosteroids improves and accelerate patients' healing. Long-term results about conventional therapies versus corticosteroids are comparable; due to understandable considering that adhesive capsulitis is a self-limiting pathology.

Another possible application of corticosteroids involves infiltration within the subacromial bursa; this method is particularly useful in those cases of acute painful bursitis, in combination with other therapies aimed at treating the underlying cause.

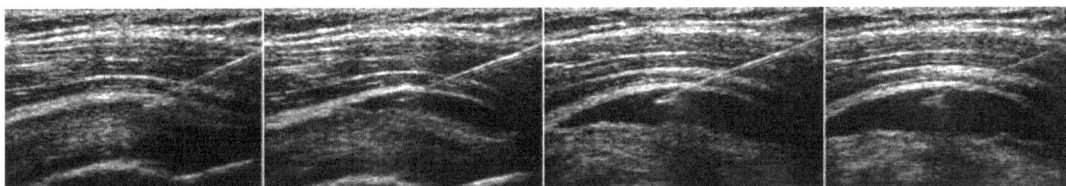

Sequence of subacromial bursa infiltration.

Besides the corticosteroids, whose action and effectiveness are widely dealt in literature, the use of the viscosupplementation with hyaluronic acid is becoming increasingly widespread. Hyaluronic acid acts through different mechanisms when injected into the joint. It is an anionic, nonsulfated glycosaminoglycan distributed widely throughout connective, epithelial and neural tissues, is capable of retaining water and this contributes to cell adhesion, proliferation and migration. High local concentrations cause the release of growth factors, accelerating the tissue repair process. The viscosupplementation is a way to restore rheological properties of the synovial fluid, enhancing viscoelastic properties of synovial fluid protecting cartilage from mechanical stress and reducing pain.

In the tendinitis involving the rotator cuff, viscosupplementation, not only protects the joint surface, but also restores the homeostasis of the chondrocytes. The hypothesis that hyaluronic acid also acts on pain modulation has been investigated and Mitsui demonstrate that hyaluronic acid inhibits not only expression of mRNA for proinflammatory cytokines, such as IL-1b, IL-6 and TNF-a, but also COX-2/PGE2 (Prostaglandin E2) production via CD44 in IL-1-stimulated subacromial-synovium fibroblasts. CD44 is also present on synoviocytes, so it is a target for pain reduction. The restoration of the viscoelastic barrier around the nociceptive afferent fibers, reduces pain, hindering interaction with nociceptive stimuli.

Rehabilitation

The rehabilitation program should always start from clinical evaluation, focusing on the status of functional deficiency, the range of motion and the pain elicited during evaluation. The aim is to ensure long-term results in joint mobility, to reduce stiffness and improve function.

Maintaining the range of movements is essential to prevent adhesion and decrease impingement. To intervene on the strength of the rotator cuff muscles and on the scapula stabilizing muscles (anterior serratus, rhomboids, latissimus dorsi and trapezium) and the deltoid, avoids the superior migration of the humeral head and the scapular instability, two conditions that occur in the impingement syndrome.

A deficit in neuromuscular control may cause abnormalities in the rotator cuff and scapula-thoracic muscles. It has been postulated that proprioception can modulate the sensitivity of muscle spindles and help subjects to pay more attention to joint position.

Exercises that specifically generate higher level of activation of the rotator cuff, lower trapezius or serratus anterior, are open-chain exercises included full can, side lying external rotation, diagonal exercise and prone full can at 100° of abduction. While the closed-chain exercises facilitate the co-contraction of shoulder muscles as well as strengthen the serratus anterior.

The brain guides motion tasks by interacting with external signals and proprioceptive stimuli. Therefore, stimuli integration takes place here and the center that generates an answer to them can be re-edited.

A possible way to reach this aim is the Multi-Joint System (MJS), a system consisting of a multi-articulated arm run by the patient on the three planes of space. The patient receives feedback from a computer system connected to the robot arm and adjusts his movements, following predefined trajectories. In this way, the patient learns to perform all the peculiar movements of the glenohumeral joint, maintaining a proper position of the scapula and increasing the strength of the anterior serratus, rhomboid, latissimus dorsi, trapezius and deltoid. MJS grant a better control of shoulder movements with increased proprioception, sensitivity and shoulder joint motion in a multi-dimensional axial-type range.

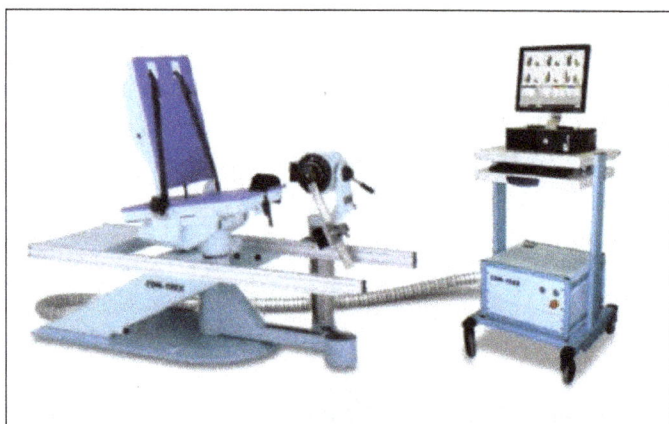

Multi-Joint System.

Low Back Pain

Low back pain (LBP) has become an increasing problem around the world. It is increasing as a result of an ageing and expanding world population. The years lived with disability from low back pain have gone up by more than 50% since 1990, particularly in low-income and middle-income countries. In general, it is related to smoking, obesity, sedentary occupations, and to low socioeconomic status (with poor quality of life and limited resources). In low-income and middle-income countries, disability and costs from low back pain will rise in the future, especially where health systems are delicate and cannot cope with this increasing burden. Globally, in 2016, low back pain contributed 57.6 million [95% uncertainty interval (UI) 40.8–75.9 million (7.2%, 6.0–8.3)] of total years lived with disability (YLDs).

The cultural, social, and political environment of back pain can influence the perception of pain, the disability created, and the use of health care. High-quality economic appraisals of looking at surgery when compared to conservative care (with the use of different treatment options) are needed in chronic low back pain (CLBP) patients.

Guidelines recommend the non-pharmacological and non-invasive management. These include the provision of advice to stay active and the use of patient education and exercise therapy]. Guidelines regularly recommend the use of physical exercise for non-specific LBP. Guidelines endorse the cautious use of imaging, of medication, and of surgery. A risk stratification tool is recommended in the National Institute for Health and Care Excellence (NICE) guidelines, so that treatments can be co-ordinated to each risk subgroup.

Patients with low back pain can be triaged using a clinical assessment. This should include history-taking, physical examination, and neurological tests to recognize radicular features. With low back pain, patients should be screened for 'red flags' to exclude serious pathologies, and diagnostic tests (such as imaging) carried out if suspected.

Psychosocial risk factors (yellow flags using prognostic screening tools) should be assessed to predict poorer outcomes. There can be mutual decisions made with the patient as to whether simpler and less-intensive management is called for. If there is no improvement after 4 weeks, and a serious pathology or radiculopathy is suspected, then specialist consultation is recommended.

Examples of simpler management include guidance and reassurance on self-management, guidance to stay active and avoid bed rest, guidance to return to normal activities, or referral for a group or an individual exercise program. This could be combined with manual or psychological therapies in a combined rehabilitation programme.

Prevention

Public health programs that challenge obesity and low physical activity levels should be developed and provide the forum for decreasing the effects of low back pain on daily living. In CLBP, evidence for prevention and treatment often comes from high-income countries. Whether or not these guideline recommendations are applicable for low-income and middle-income countries, remains unknown. Public health programs and their urgency will differ in high-income countries when compared to low-income and middle-income countries as well. An obstacle in altering health pathways concerns the existing models of health-care reimbursement. It is useful to have the whole health pathway for low back pain mapped out, from the first contact all the way through to specialized care.

Health-care professionals should deliver regular education concerning the causes, the mechanisms, the natural history, and prognosis of low back pain, and promote the benefits of physical activity and exercise.

Exercise alone or in combination with education has shown moderate-quality evidence that this is effective for prevention of LBP. Its preventive effect was found to be high, with a pooled relative risk of 0.55 (95% CI 0.41–0.74). With intensive programs, exercise then can be focused on secondary prevention.

In 2014, a systematic study and meta-analysis found only four pediatric trials in pediatric low back pain. This casts doubt regarding the evidence for treatment of back pain in children. There was moderate-quality evidence that education was not effective in children. There was very low quality evidence that ergonomically designed furniture prevented low back pain.

A recent meta-analysis was performed on the prevention of low back pain using exercise. Exercise on its own was able to decrease the risk of LBP by 33% (risk ratio = 0.67; 95% CI 0.53, 0.85, I^2 = 23%, where I^2 describes the percentage of variation across studies that is due to heterogeneity rather than chance; eight randomized controlled trials; n = 1634). When exercise was combined with education, it reduced the risk by 27% (risk ratio = 0.73; 95% CI 0.59, 0.91, I^2 = 6%; six trials; n = 1381). The intensity of LBP and the accompanying disability from LBP were also decreased in the exercise groups when compared to the control groups. The analysis concluded that exercise diminished the risk of LBP and its associated disability. A mixture of strengthening with either stretching or aerobic exercises when performed two to three times per week could sensibly be endorsed for the prevention of LBP in the general population.

Management of Acute Low Back Pain

For acute non-specific low back pain that does not have serious pathology (red flags have been excluded), initial reassurance, advice to stay active and self-management are all that is needed. Self-management can include self-exercises and education from reading booklets or being involved in on-line education for low back pain.

Table: Management of acute low back pain (without serious pathology).

Acute low back pain (without serious pathology)
Initial reassurance, guidance to stay active and avoid bed rest, and provide guidance on self-management.
Self-management can include self-exercises and education from reading booklets or being involved in online education for low back pain.
Primary conservative physical treatment may include exercises, superficial heat, and manual therapy.
Guidance to return to normal activities, or referral for an individual or group exercise program.
Pharmacological therapies include nonsteroidal anti-inflammatory drugs (NSAIDs) and weak opioids for brief periods (paracetamol is not recommended).
Progress should be reviewed in 7–14 days.

Recommended primary conservative physical treatment preferences include manual therapy, exercise, and superficial heat. There is low evidence that low-level laser therapy is more effective than sham laser for pain. Limited evidence shows that acupuncture is modestly effective for acute low back pain. The McKenzie method of mechanical diagnosis and therapy (MDT) is designed to categorize patients into homogeneous subgroups (derangement, dysfunction, or postural syndrome. This is in order to direct treatment with specific exercises and postural advice. In acute LBP, moderate- to high-quality evidence exists that MDT is not superior to other rehabilitation interventions in decreasing pain and disability. Back schools use varying exercises and educational methods. There is very low-quality evidence that back school is more effective than no treatment (mean difference (MD) – 6.10, 95% confidence interval (CI) – 10.18 to – 2.01) in acute low back pain.

In acute low back pain, when pharmacological therapies are considered, these would include nonsteroidal anti-inflammatory drugs (NSAIDs), skeletal muscle relaxants, and weak opioids for brief periods (paracetamol is not recommended).

For acute low back pain, most patients improve with or without therapy. The magnitude of pain benefits is small to moderate and generally short term. Progress should be reviewed in 7–14 days. Guidance should be given to return to normal activities, or referral made for an individual or group exercise program.

There has been no recommendation as to the level of pain allowed during exercise, and to the level of pain tolerated at each stage of the exercise progression. A systematic study protocol has recently been published in order to study the effect of using a differentiation of exercises based on the amount of low back pain experienced by patients in primary care.

The guidelines recommend early non-pharmacological treatment that includes education and self-management, and the recommencement of normal activities and exercise, with the addition of psychological programs in those whose symptoms persist.

Physical Treatment Preferences

In low back pain, guidelines promote the avoidance of bed rest, and the continuation with activities as usual. The aim of physical treatments is to improve function, and to prevent disability from getting worse. In chronic low back pain, exercise therapy has become a first-line treatment and should be routinely used.

Should recovery be slow in patients with risk factors for developing persistent disabling pain, early supervised exercise therapy can be considered. If low back pain persists for more than 12 weeks, physical treatments that encompass a graded activity or exercise programs that focus on improvements in function, are recommended. In fact, in low back pain greater than 12 weeks, exercise is a first-line treatment that should be considered for routine use. All recent clinical practice guidelines endorse exercise therapy in persistent low back pain. Yet access to structured exercise programs remains erratic.

In clinical practice guidelines, there remain large inconsistencies in the type of exercise program (yoga, stretching, hydrotherapy exercises, tai chi, McKenzie exercise approach and back schools) needed, and in the way that it is delivered (group exercise individual programs, or supervised home exercise). Choice may ultimately depend on patients' preferences and on the experience of the treating therapist. Clinical practice guidelines now suggest that a diversity of types of exercises should be used. Exercise induces pain relief by the activation of central inhibitory paths. Mechanisms involving opioids, serotonin, and N-methyl-d-aspartate (NMDA) in the rostral ventromedial medulla stimulates pain relief associated with exercise.

Back pain prevalence is low in children, but increases during adolescence. A systematic study has found that prevention and treatment interventions having an exercise component are most likely to be effective.

There is no evidence available to show that one type of exercise is superior to another. In deciding on the type of exercise to be used, guidelines should, however, incorporate individual preferences, needs, and capabilities. Movement control tests, laterality judgment, and two-point discrimination show the highest level of known-groups validity for people with chronic low back pain. Nonetheless, the reliability of these measurement tools has yet to be established.

In chronic low back without serious pathology, recommended primary conservative physical treatment preferences include exercise, yoga, biofeedback, progressive relaxation, massage, manual therapy, and interdisciplinary rehabilitation.

Table: Management of chronic low back pain (without serious pathology).

Chronic low back pain (without serious pathology)
Triage using a clinical assessment (history-taking, physical examination, and neurological tests (to recognize radicular features).
Patients should be screened for 'red flags' to exclude serious pathologies, and diagnostic tests (such as imaging) only carried out if suspected.
Patients should be screened for psychosocial risk factors ('yellow flags' such as low self-efficacy, catastrophizing, fear of movement) to predict poorer outcomes.
Use a risk stratification tool (such as STarT).

Non-pharmacological and non-invasive management treatment is recommended that includes education and self-management, and the recommencement of normal activities and exercise, with the addition of psychological programs in those whose symptoms persist (multidisciplinary treatments).
Primary conservative physical treatment exercises include walking, Pilates, tai chi, yoga, progressive relaxation (and massage, and manual therapy in some guidelines).
No evidence available to show that one type of exercise is superior to another Choice may ultimately depend on patients' preferences and on the experience of the treating therapist. A diversity of types of exercises should be used.
Physical therapy exercise approach remains a first-line treatment, and should routinely be used Referral could be for an individual or group exercise program Passive physical therapies (massage, spinal mobilization, acupuncture, and spinal manipulation with radiculopathy) are not usually endorsed, or are optional in some guidelines.
Passive methods (rest, medications) are associated with worsening disability, and are not recommended.
Pharmacological therapies if used include nonsteroidal anti-inflammatory drugs (NSAIDs) and antidepressants at the lowest effective dose and for the least possible time.
Injections, denervation procedures, and the use of surgery are generally not endorsed.
No improvement after 4 weeks, or pathology or radiculopathy suspected, then specialist consultation.

In spinal pain with radiculopathy, exercise and spinal manipulation can be used. However, some guidelines do not endorse the use of passive therapies, or make them optional in patients unresponsive to other treatments. These include massage, spinal manipulation or mobilization, and acupuncture.

Other passive physical or electrical methods, such as short-wave diathermy, interferential therapy transcutaneous electrical nerve stimulation (TENS), back supports, traction, and ultrasound have been largely found to be ineffective, and are not recommended. A systematic study has shown that high-quality randomized controlled trials (RCTs) to determine the effects of TENS are needed due to the low quality of present studies, wherein adequate parameters and timing of assessment were not consistently reported or used.

Association with Psychosocial Factors

In the treatment of back pain by physiotherapists, an association exists with psychosocial factors, such as self-efficacy, catastrophizing, fear of movement, and pain and disability outcomes. A recent systematic study looked at the psychosocial factors related to change in pain and disability outcomes in chronic low back pain patients that were treated by physiotherapists. An association was found between psychosocial factors, such as self-efficacy, catastrophizing, and fear of movement, and pain and disability outcomes.

Pilates

An exercise system centering on controlled movement, breathing, and stretching is known as Pilates. Most clinical trials in the past 5 years have found Pilates to be an effective rehabilitation tool that has resulted in desired outcomes, such as reducing pain and disability.

Yoga

A Cochrane systematic study demonstrated a slight functional improvement when yoga is used for chronic non-specific low back pain with a slight reduction in pain; it heightened the chance of clinical improvement. In some people, however, it was found to increase their back pain.

Walking

The advantage of walking is that it is easy to carry out. In chronic low back pain, a meta-analysis of nine suitable randomized controlled trials was performed to understand the effectiveness of walking on disability, pain, and quality of life at post intervention and at follow-up visits. The duration of follow-up, namely: short-term (< 3 months), intermediate-term (between 3 and 12 months), and long-term (> 12 months), was used to analyze the data. In short- and intermediate-term follow-ups, walking was found (with low- to moderate-quality evidence) to be as effective as other non-pharmacological interventions in decreasing disability and pain, and was recommended.

Mobilization and Manipulation Therapies

A recent systematic literature study and meta-analysis has examined mobilization and manipulation for treating chronic low back pain. Bias was assessed using the Scottish Intercollegiate Guidelines Network criteria. The confidence in effect estimates was defined using the Grading of Recommendations, Assessment, Development, and Evaluation (GRADE) system. Nine trials (1176 patients) provided sufficient data. Following treatment, the standardized mean difference for a decrease in pain was standardized mean difference (SMD) = -0.28, [95% confidence interval (CI) -0.47 to -0.09, $p = 0.004$; $I^2 = 57\%$ (where I^2 describes the percentage of variation across studies that is due to heterogeneity rather than chance)]. When mobilization or manipulation was compared to other active therapies, seven trials (923 patients) showed the decrease in disability to be a SMD = -0.33, [95% CI -0.63 to -0.03, $p = 0.03$; $I^2 = 78\%$].

Subgroup analyses showed that mobilization when compared to other active comparators (that included exercise), significantly decreased pain (SMD = -0.20, [95% CI -0.35 to -0.04; $p = 0.01$; $I^2 = 0\%$]), but not disability (SMD = -0.10, [95% CI -0.28 to 0.07; $p = 0.25$; $I^2 = 21\%$].

Subgroup analyses showed that manipulation when compared to other active comparators (that included physical therapy and exercise), significantly decreased pain and disability (SMD = -0.43, [95% CI -0.86 to 0.00; $p = 0.05$, $I^2 = 79\%$; SMD = -0.86, 95% CI -1.27 to -0.45; $p < 0.0001$, $I^2 = 46\%$], respectively).

A systematic study and meta-analysis of manipulation and mobilization in the treatment of chronic low back pain published in 2018, found moderate-quality evidence that manipulation and mobilization decreased pain and increased function. Manipulation seemed to be more effective than mobilization, although both were safe.

Movement Control Exercises

A systematic study and meta-analysis of the effectiveness of movement control exercise on patients with non-specific low back pain and movement control impairment (MVCE), was recently carried out. There was 'very low to moderate quality evidence of a positive effect of MVCE on disability, both at the end of treatment (SMD -0.38; 95% CI -0.68, -0.09), and after 12 months (SMD 0.37; 95% CI -0.61, -0.04). Pain intensity became significantly decreased after MVCE at the end of treatment (SMD -0.39; 95% CI -0.69, -0.04), but not after 12 months (SMD -0.27; 95% CI -0.62, 0.09).

Technology-supported Exercise Therapy

Technological systems, such as electromyography feedback (EMG-FB) provide technology-supported exercise therapy (TSET), and have been progressed to benefit exercise therapy for low back pain. In patients with low back pain, a recent systematic study found that TSET improved pain, disability, and quality of life. However, for most technologies, only a limited number of RCTs were available, and solid conclusions regarding the effectiveness of individual technological systems could not be made.

McKenzie Method of Mechanical Diagnosis and Therapy

Using the information obtained from the McKenzie Method of Mechanical Diagnosis and Therapy (MDT) assessment, the clinician will then prescribe specific exercises and advice regarding postures to adopt and postures to temporarily avoid. A recent literature study with meta-analysis in patients with chronic LBP found moderate- to high-quality evidence that MDT was superior to other rehabilitation interventions in reducing pain and disability, but was dependent on the type of intervention used for comparison to MDT.

Pregnancy

Another meta-analysis found that even during and after pregnancy, osteopathic manipulative treatment for low back and pelvic girdle pain during and after pregnancy gave clinically relevant benefits. A meta-analysis of randomized controlled trials (RCTs) published in 2018 showed that exercise decreased the risk of low back pain in pregnancy by 9% [pooled risk ratio (RR) = 0.91; 95% CI 0.83–0.99; I^2 = 0%, seven trials; n = 1175]. However, there was no protective effect on pelvic girdle pain (RR = 0.99; CI 0.81–1.21; I^2 = 0%; four RCTs; n = 565), or on lumbar- pelvic pain (RR = 0.96; CI 0.90–1.02; I^2 = 0%; eight RCTs; n = 1737). In lumbar-pelvic pain, exercise was able to prevent new episodes of sick leave (RR = 0.79; CI 0.64–0.99; I^2 = 0%; three RCTs; n = 1168).

Knee Injury

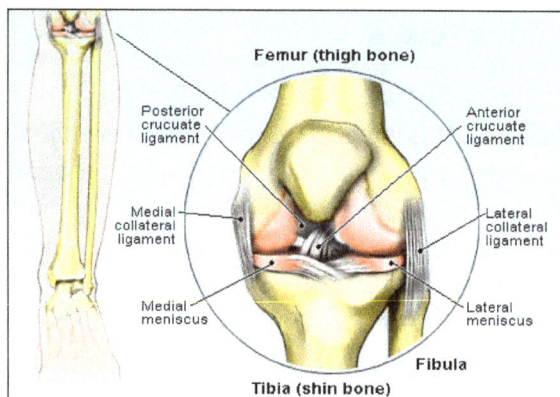

The knee is one of the most common body parts to be injured. Types of common knee injuries include sprains, strains, bursitis, dislocations, fractures, meniscus tears, and overuse injuries.

Knee injuries are generally caused by twisting or bending force applied to the knee, or a direct blow, such as from sports, falls, or accidents. Risk factors for knee injury include overuse, improper training, having osteoporosis, and playing high-impact sports that involve sudden changes in direction. The main signs and symptoms of knee injury are knee painand swelling.

Knee injuries are diagnosed by a history and physical examination. Sometimes an X-ray or MRI may be done. Treatment of knee injuries depends on the type and severity of the injury and can involve RICE therapy (rest, ice, compression, elevation), physical therapy, immobilization, or surgery.

Prognosis for knee injury depends on the type and severity of the injury and the need for physical therapy or surgery. Prevention of knee pain and injuries involves proper training, proper equipment, and maintaining a safe playing field or home environment to avoid falls.

What are the Different Types of Knee Injuries?

The knee is one of the most commonly injured parts of the body. Sports, falls, and motor-vehicle accidents account for the vast majority of knee pain and injuries to the knee.

The different types of common knee injuries to the knee are defined by the affected anatomy of the knee and the mechanism by which it's injured.

Knee sprains are injuries to the ligaments that hold the knee together. There are multiple ligaments that stabilize the knee and keep it in alignment. The anterior cruciate ligament (ACL) and the posterior cruciate ligament (PCL) stabilize the knee in movement from front to back and cross each other in the middle of the knee joint. The medial collateral ligament (MCL) and lateral collateral ligament (LCL) stabilize the knee so that the bones do not slide from side to side.

Ligament sprains are graded by the amount of stretching or tearing of the ligament fibers and how much instability it causes as follows:

- Grade 1 knee sprain: The ligament is stretched and painful, but fibers are not torn and no instability is present.

- Grade 2 knee sprain: The ligament fibers are torn partially, mild instability may be evident.

- Grade 3 knee sprain: The ligament fibers are completely torn and the knee is unstable.

Knee strains occur when tendons or muscles surrounding the knee are stretched, usually due to hyperflexion or hyperextension of the knee. These strains can lead to pain outside of the knee joint but can cause dysfunction of the normal range of motion of the knee. The patellar tendon stretches from the lower kneecap to the front of the tibia bone at the front of the leg.

Knee bursitis occurs when a fluid-filled pouch (called a bursa) in the knee is irritated, inflamed, or infected. Bursas are fluid-filled sacs located around joints that act as shock absorbers that minimize the friction between various tissues, such as the muscles and tendons around the joints. In the knee, there are two main bursas, one above the kneecap (patella), and one below the knee joint near the front of the tibia bone.

Tears of the meniscus can occur from damage to the inside of the knee. The medial and lateral menisci (plural of meniscus) are semi-round, articular cartilage that act as shock absorbers and smooth cushions for the thighbone (femur). These menisci can be injured acutely or can become dysfunctional gradually due to overuse and/or aging.

Knee joint dislocation can occur due to high-impact, large-force injuries to the knee (sports, motor vehicle accidents). This is a rare injury but causes severe damage to all the anatomical components of the knee and can include damage to the blood vessels and nerves about the knee. This requires emergency treatment or surgery.

The kneecap (patella) can dislocate to the side of the knee. Patellar dislocation can be very painful but is generally not life-threatening and can be treated by popping it back into place (reduction of the patella), splinting, and physical therapy.

Knee fractures occur from direct blows to the bones. Patella, or kneecap, fractures occur when a person falls directly down onto the knees and the kneecap cracks due to the force. Collapse of the top of the tibia bone in the knee (tibia plateau fracture) can occur from sudden compression injury to the knee, especially in people with osteoporosis.

Other fractures of the long bones (fibula, tibia, and femur) are rare with isolated injures to the knee.

Other overuse injuries of the knee include patellofemoral pain syndrome (often referred to as "runner's knee," which causes pain on the front of the knee) and weakness and degeneration of the cartilage under the kneecap (chondromalacia patella). These injuries are due to an accumulation of repetitive damage to the knee structures. Congenital knee problems or improper mechanics of the knee movement may cause this.

Osteochondritis dissecans is a joint disorder that occurs most commonly in children. Bone and cartilage beneath the joints loses its blood supply, resulting in joint pain and stiffness. This condition typically affects the knees, but it can also affect other joints such as elbows and ankles.

Osgood-Schlatter disease is a condition in children caused by growth spurts that cause knee pain and swelling below the kneecap.

What Causes a Knee Injury?

Most knee injuries are caused by an external force bending or twisting the knee in a manner that it was not anatomically designed for. Common causes of knee injuries are from a twisting mechanism from falls, sports, or accidents. A twisted knee can cause damage to the ligaments and cartilage.

High-force injuries such as sports-related injuries and motor vehicle accidents can disrupt multiple parts of the knee anatomy, causing multiple types of knee injuries.

Bursitis can be caused by overuse, arthritis, degenerative joint disease, injuries from kneeling, infection, or gout.

What are Risk Factors for a Knee Injury?

High-impact sports, including running, basketball, football, hockey, soccer, cycling, and others, can increase the risk of knee pain and injury. Sports where shoes with cleats are worn and sharp, sudden changes in direction are made, along with contact sports, are common risks for knee injury. Exercise, such as high-impact cardiovascular activity or yoga, can also cause knee injury. The elderly may be at higher risk for knee injury due to falls and osteoporosis.

Women may be at higher risk for anterior cruciate ligament injuries (ACL) and patellar injuries. This is due to the anatomy of a woman's hips and femur and the angle at which the knee is tilted. This can lead to chondromalacia patella (CMP), an inflammation or irritation of the underside of the patella.

Being overweight can be a risk factor for knee injury, as excess weight puts more stress on the lower extremity joints.

Overuse and overtraining, improper or insufficient training for a sport, or not properly rehabilitating acute injuries can also predispose a person to knee injuries.

Physical therapy for knee pain involves a thorough evaluation and assessment of your entire lower extremity from your hip to your foot. Your PT can assess your knee pain and prescribe the right treatments — including exercises and modalities — to help decrease your knee pain and improve your overall mobility.

Anatomy of the Knee

The human knee is a hinge joint that is comprised of the tibia (shin) and the femur (thigh). The patella, or kneecap, is located in the front of the knee. The knee is supported by four ligaments. Two shock absorbers, each called a meniscus, are found within the knee.

Pain in the knee can be caused by repetitive trauma and strain or injury. Occasionally it occurs for no apparent reason. When knee pain occurs, you may experience functional limitations that include difficulty walking, rising from sitting, or ascending and descending stairs.

What Type of Knee Pain do you have?

If you experience knee pain, it is important to determine if the pain is acute, sub-acute, or chronic in nature. This can help guide proper diagnosis and treatment.

- Acute Pain: Usually the most severe and occurs 1-7 days after injury. During this time, you should rest the knee and let the injured structures heal before initiating any motion.

- Sub-Acute Pain: This occurs from 2-6 weeks after injury. This is a good time to initiate gentle motion around the knee to help regain mobility.

- Chronic Knee Pain: Pain lasting greater than 8-12 weeks. Knee pain that is chronic should be evaluated by your healthcare provider.

Location of Knee Pain Symptoms

The location of your knee pain can help determine which structures are at fault and can help ensure proper treatment. Remember to check with your physician, physical therapist, or healthcare provider if symptoms are severe or last more than a few weeks.

- Pain in the Front of the Knee: If you feel pain in the front of the knee, there may be a problem with the tracking and position of the kneecap, often called patellofemoral stress syndrome (PFSS). The kneecap and the tendon between the kneecap and the shin may become inflamed and painful. Pain here usually limits the ability to kneel, ascend or descend stairs, or run and jump.

- Pain on the Inside of the Knee: If you have pain on the inside portion of the knee, there is likely an injury to the medial meniscus or medial collateral ligament. These structures are usually injured during athletic activity when the foot is planted on the ground, and the body twists over the knee. The medial meniscus is a shock absorber located inside the knee. Occasionally, it suffers from wear and tear or arthritis and can be damaged with no specific injury.

- Pain on the Outside of the Knee: Pain on the outside aspect of your knee can be the result of injury to many structures. There is a ligament there that may be injured during athletic activity. Pain here can also be caused by iliotibial band (ITB) stress. The ITB is a thick band of tissue that runs from the outside of your hip to the front of your knee. As it crosses the knee, the ITB can rub abnormally on the knee, and a burning pain can ensue. Also, on the outside part of the knee is one of the three hamstring tendons. Strain to this tendon may be a source of knee pain.

- Pain in the Back of the Knee: Pain in the back of the knee is rare but can occur. One of the hamstring tendons attaches here, and pain here is likely due to a hamstring strain. Another possible cause of pain here is a Baker's cyst. This is an abnormal swelling of the knee joint that occupies space in the back of the knee and causes pain with excessive bending of the knee.

If you develop acute knee pain, immediately follow the R.I.C.E. principle. R.I.C.E. stands for Rest, Ice, Compression, and Elevation. After a few days of R.I.C.E., you can begin using the leg, only gently.

What to Expect from Physical Therapy for Knee Pain

If you are referred to physical therapy for knee pain, the initial visit is important to ensure correct diagnosis and proper management. During this visit, your physical therapist will interview you to gather information about the history of your problem, about the aggravating and relieving factors, and about any past medical history that may contribute the overall problem. From the information gathered during the history, a focused examination will be conducted. The examination may consist of several sections including, but not limited to:

- Gait Evaluation: An assessment of how you are walking. Physical therapists are trained to notice small changes in the motion around the knee during different phases of walking.

- Palpation: This involves using the hands to touch various structures around the knee to feel for abnormalities or to assess if a structure is painful to touch.

- Range of Motion Measurements: Range of motion refers to how far the knee is bending or straightening. The physical therapist may use special instruments to measure how your knee is moving to help direct treatment.

- Strength Measurements: There are many muscular attachments around the knee, and a measurement of strength can help determine if muscular weakness or imbalance is causing your knee pain.

- Assessment of Your Balance: If your balance is impaired, excessive stress and strain may be directed to your knee and cause pain.

- Girth or Swelling Measurements: Occasionally, swelling may be present in the knee joint after injury. A physical therapist may measure the amount of swelling to help direct treatment.

- Special Tests: Special tests are specific maneuvers performed around the knee to help determine which structure may be at fault and may be causing the problem.

PT Treatment for Knee Pain

After a focused examination has been completed, your physical therapist can work with you to initiate the correct treatment. It is very important for you to be active and engaged in the program. Often, exercises to help strengthen and improve the mobility of the knee will be prescribed. You may be required to perform exercises at home as well as part of a home exercise program.

Exercise should be your main tool for treating your knee pain. Exercises to help your knee pain may include:

- Quad sets and straight leg raises.

- Short arc quads.

- Exercises to strengthen your hips (Your hip muscles help control the position of your knees. Weakness here may cause knee pain).

- Lower extremity stretches.

- Balance exercises.

Your PT will tell you how often to perform your exercises at home, and he or she should monitor your progress when you visit the PT clinic. He or she may also perform other treatments while you are in the PT clinic. These may include:

- Ultrasound.

- Electric stimulation.

- Kinesiology taping.

- Application of heat or ice.

- Soft tissue massages or knee joint mobilization.

Keep in mind that passive treatments like ultrasound or estim have not been proven to be the most effective treatment for knee pain. They may feel good, but your focus with PT should be on restoring functional mobility. You should discuss the overall goal of each treatment so you have an understanding of what to expect.

If knee pain persists for more than two to three weeks or occurs as the result of major trauma, a visit to a physician or health care provider is recommended.

Parkinson's Disease

Parkinson's disease is a progressive, degenerative clinical condition that worsens over time. Typical symptoms include tremors, loss of facial expression, stiffness, slowing down of movement and a multitude of other problems.

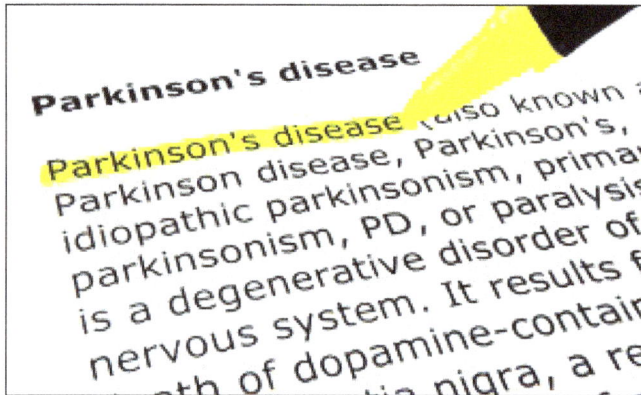

In the past few years, there have been significant developments in the understanding of Parkinson's disease. Treatment includes a combination of medication, diet, exercise, lifestyle modifications, counseling and participation in support groups.

Physical Therapy can Help

Parkinson's disease is associated with the inability to produce the chemical dopamine in the brain. Dopamine is a chemical messenger that transmits information between brain cells. The reduction of dopamine causes symptoms such as tremors (typically described as 'pill rolling'), tightening of the muscles (called rigidity) and slowing down of movements (called hypokinesia). These features can cause a great deal of disability, and can be effectively managed with physical therapy.

Advice for Caregivers

Since there is no known cure, the objective of physical therapy in Parkinson's disease is to slow down the degenerative effects of this disease as much as possible.

Parkinson's disease affects each individual in a different way. A physical therapist will work closely with the patient and family members to monitor the condition and improve functional capacity as much as possible. This is a life-altering event and caregivers or family members may react with denial, confusion, fear, anger, or self-blame.

The physical therapist will conduct an evaluation of gait, balance, coordination, strength and posture of the patient. The caregiver is provided the tools and information to keep the patient mobile with movement patterns and home exercise programs.

Depending upon the severity and nature of the patient's condition, the treatment plan focuses on the following:

- Developing an effective strategy to get in and out of bed and maintain balance in sitting and standing.

- Improving endurance, strength, and flexibility.

- Enhancing dexterity to perform hand movements.

- Maintaining coordination while walking and changing directions.

- Decreasing risk of falls.

- Ascending and descending stairs.

- Managing multiple tasks simultaneously.

- Participating in day-to-day activities.

In the early phase, physical therapy helps maintain activity and reduce the risk of falling. Group activities like dance classes provide a refreshing way to explore movement and music.

Over a period of time, the goal is to stimulate muscle activities and preserve existing function. As the disease progresses, patients may be confined to a bed or a wheel chair. Treatment is now focused towards maintaining vital bodily function. Walking aids like a cane or walker may be prescribed.

Anxiety and despair is common when dealing with a progressive condition with no known cure. Despite the complexity of the condition, the benefits of physical therapy are significant. Helping a patient cope with disability and dysfunction from a physical and emotional perspective is the foundation of physical therapy treatment for every condition, including one as progressive as Parkinson's.

References

- The-role-of-physical-medicine-and-rehabilitation-in-shoulder-disorders, advances-in-shoulder-surgery: intechopen.com, Retrieved 08 January, 2019

- Physical-therapy-for-knee-pain-2696411: verywellhealth.com, Retrieved 14 February, 2019

- Role-of-physical-therapy-on-parkinsons-disease-treatment: starspt.org, Retrieved 16 June, 2019

- Lumbar-zygapophyseal-joint-arthropathy: now.aapmr.org, Retrieved 26 January, 2019

- Guillain-Barre-Syndrome: physio-pedia.com, Retrieved 25 August, 2019

Chapter 6

Rehabilitation of Sport-related Injuries

Physical medicine and rehabilitation play an important role in the area of sports nutrition. This chapter delves into rehabilitation of ankle and foot injuries in athletes, sports concussion, shin-splint syndrome, overhead athlete's elbow, hip and groin pain, hamstring injury, etc. to provide an extensive understanding of the subject.

Common Sports Injuries

Hip Flexor Strain

The hip flexors are muscles found on the upper-front side of your thigh. The main functions of the hip flexor muscles are to lift the knee toward your trunk, as well as assist moving your leg toward and away from the other leg. Hip flexors can be weak in individuals who sit a great deal at work or can become weak and stiff in individuals who have poor sitting posture. Sports injuries to this muscle group can be caused by sprinting, running inclines and activities with quick turns and sudden starts.

"Common symptoms of a hip flexor strain would include pain with raising the leg, such as stair climbing and transfers in and out of a car, as well as cutting and running activities," "Someone who experiences a hip flexor strain might notice bruising in the front of the upper thigh and groin area."

A hip flexor strain is best treated by rest and icing for 15 to 20 minutes at a time for the first 48 to 72 hours. After the first three recovery days, the injured athlete could apply heat for 15 to 20 minutes followed by lying down and performing gentle heel slides and hip flexor stretches. If the pain, symptoms and limited activity remain after two weeks, the individual should seek out physical therapy for pain and swelling control and instruction in specific hip-strengthening exercises to regain power, range of motion and movement.

ACL Tear or Strain

The ACL, anterior cruciate ligament, is one of the major stabilizing ligaments of the knee. The most common cause of sports injuries for an ACL strain is slowing down and trying to cut, pivot or change directions. Ligaments on the inside of the knee are often torn with the ACL injury, making it a devastating event.

Complaints of instability when walking or turning corners, as well as increased swelling in the knee would be common ACL tear symptoms. A slight ACL strain or tear can be healed without surgery using rest and ice, as the scar tissue helps heal the ligament and the knee becomes more stable. A complete ACL tear would require surgery and a few months of recovery time with aggressive physical therapy before the athlete would be able to return to activity.

Concussion

A concussion can be defined as injury to the brain, due a blow to the head where the brain is jarred or shaken. Concussions are serious injuries that should not be taken lightly. An athlete who experiences a concussion should seek out a certified athletic trainer or a physician with experience treating concussions. Common concussion symptoms can include:

- Headache,

- Confusion,

- Dizziness,

- Nausea and/or vomiting,

- Slurred speech,

- Sensitivity to light,

- Delayed response to questions.

Athletes diagnosed with a concussion should never return to their sport without being medically cleared by a health care professional trained in concussion evaluation.

Common concussion treatments include rest, reduced activities requiring mental or physical stress and slowly increasing physical activities, as long as symptoms do not return.

Groin Pull

A groin pull is also called a groin strain. The groin muscles run from the upper-inner thigh to the inner thigh right above the knee. Groin muscles pull the legs together and are often injured with quick side-to-side movements and/or a lack of flexibility. The injured athlete might notice difficulty with lateral movements, getting in and out of cars, as well as tenderness or bruising in the groin or inner thigh.

Groin pull treatment includes rest and icing for 15 to 20 minutes periodically during the first 72 hours. After the first three days, the athlete could use heat for 15 to 20 minutes periodically, followed by gentle, proper groin stretching and range of motion exercises, for example, by making snow angels on the floor.

Shin Splints

Athletes with shin splints complain of pain in the lower leg bone, or the tibia. Shin splints are most often found in athletes who are runners or participate in activities with a great deal of running, such as soccer. Athletes typically get shin splints diagnosed early in their season, as they increase activities or mileage too quickly. Shin splints are best prevented and/or treated with rest, icing and gradually increasing running activities. Purchasing shoes with good arch support can also reduce pain in the shins and help with recovery.

Sciatica

Sciatica is back pain that also travels down the back of the leg or even to the feet. This radiating pain can additionally be associated with numbness, burning and tingling down the leg. Sciatica can be seen in athletes who are in a flexed forward posture, such as cyclists, or athletes who perform a great deal of trunk rotation in the swing sports, like golf and tennis. The back pain and radiating pain can be caused by a bulging disc or a pinched nerve. Sometimes, rest, stretching the back and hamstrings and laying on your stomach can help alleviate the symptoms. If pain, numbness or tingling persists for more than two weeks, then the athlete should seek out a medical professional, such as a physical therapist, to help alleviate sciatica symptoms.

Hamstring Strain

The hamstring muscle is located on the back of the thigh. Unfortunately, the hamstring muscles can be tight and are susceptible to a strain, which is also called a pulled muscle. Poor stretching techniques or lack of stretching can be the cause of a hamstring tear/ strain. Often, an athlete with a hamstring tear will experience bruising in the back of the thigh or the knee. Rest and icing are the common early treatment techniques for a pulled hamstring, followed by gentle stretching and strengthening to prevent another injury. If the pain persists more than two weeks, the athlete could try physical therapy to use ultrasound or other methods to promote healing the pulled muscle.

Tennis or Golf Elbow

Tennis and golfer's elbow is usually seen with athletes performing a great deal of gripping activities. It can be labeled as an overuse sports injury, also known as medial or lateral epicondylitis. Due to the repetitive action, the tendons of the forearm can become inflamed and make any wrist or hand motions extremely painful. Often, athletes will complain of a lack of grip strength. Early treatment options for tennis or golf elbow involve rest and icing the inflamed area. Doctors will often prescribe anti-inflammatory medication, or even a brace, to try to take pressure off the area and prevent further elbow injuries. Stretching techniques and other strengthening exercises applied by an occupational or physical therapist can help to break down the stiffness and gradually build strength, returning athletes to their sporting activities.

Shoulder Injury

Shoulder injuries cover a large number of sports injuries from dislocations, misalignment, strains on muscles and sprains of ligaments.

The shoulder is the weakest joint of the body and is subject to a great deal of force during athletic activities. Many shoulder injuries can be caused by either a lack of flexibility, strength or stabilization.

Shoulder injury treatment starts with rest and icing to help with pain and swelling relief. Any pain persisting for more than two weeks should be evaluated by a physical therapist.

Patellofemoral Syndrome

The majority of sports injuries involve the lower body, particularly knee injuries. One of the most common knee injuries is called patellofemoral syndrome. This diagnosis can be caused by a slip or a fall onto the knees, swelling of the knee joint or a muscle imbalance. The patella, or kneecap, should travel in the groove at the end of the femur or thigh bone. Sometimes, a fall onto the knee can cause swelling, leading to a muscle imbalance of the two major muscles that aid in proper tracking of the kneecap in the groove. This muscle imbalance can create more swelling, making the tracking problem even worse. Rest and ice can help with knee injury pain and swelling. Gentle isometric, or static, strengthening exercises for the inner thigh muscle and gently stretching muscles for the outer or lateral thigh muscles can help to correct the muscle imbalance. If knee injury pain or dysfunction continues for more than two weeks, a referral to a physical therapist could help with more aggressive stretching and strengthening. A physical therapist may use knee taping or bracing techniques to aid with proper tracking.

Sports Specific Rehabilitation

Musculoskeletal injuries are an inevitable result of sport participation. Football has the highest incidence of catastrophic injuries, with gymnastics and ice hockey close behind. Tissue injury from sports can be classified as macrotraumatic and microtraumatic.

- Macrotraumatic injuries are usually due to a strong force – such as a fall, accident, collision or laceration – and are more common in contact sports such as football and rugby. These injuries can be primary (due to direct tissue damage) or secondary (due to transmission of forces or release of inflammatory mediators and other cytokinesis).

- Microtraumatic injuries are chronic injuries that result from overuse of a structure such as a muscle, joint, ligament, or tendon. This type of injury is more common in sports such as swimming, cycling and rowing.

The process of rehabilitation should start as early as possible after an injury and form a continuum with other therapeutic interventions. It can also start before or immediately after surgery when an injury requires a surgical intervention.

Rehabilitation Plan

The rehabilitation plan must take into account the fact that the objective of the patient (the athlete) is to return to the same activity and environment in which the injury occurred. Functional capacity after rehabilitation should be the same, if not better, than before injury.

The ultimate goal of the rehabilitation process is to limit the extent of the injury, reduce or reverse the impairment and functional loss, and prevent, correct or eliminate altogether the disability.

Multidisciplinary Approach

The rehabilitation of the injured athlete is managed by a multidisciplinary team with a physician functioning as the leader and coordinator of care. The team includes, but is not limited to, sports physicians, physiatrists (rehabilitation medicine practitioners), orthopaedists, physiotherapists, rehabilitation workers, physical educators, coaches, athletic trainers, psychologists, and nutritionists. The rehabilitation team works closely with the athlete and the coach to establish the rehabilitation goals, to discuss the progress resulting from the various interventions, and to establish the time frame for the return of the athletes to training and competition.

Communication is a vital factor. A lack of communication between medical providers, strength and conditioning specialists, and team coaches can slow or prevent athletes from returning to peak capability and increase the risk of new injuries and even more devastating reinjuries.

Principles

Principles are the foundation upon which rehabilitation is based. Here are seven principles of rehabilitation, which can be remembered by the mnemonic: ATC IS IT.

- A: Avoid aggravation. It is important not to aggravate the injury during the rehabilitation process. Therapeutic exercise, if administered incorrectly or without good judgment, has the potential to exacerbate the injury, that is, make it worse.

- T: Timing. The therapeutic exercise portion of the rehabilitation program should begin as soon as possible—that is, as soon as it can occur without causing aggravation. The sooner patients can begin the exercise portion of the rehabilitation program, the sooner they can return to full activity. Following injury, rest is sometimes necessary, but too much rest can actually be detrimental to recovery.

- C: Compliance. Without a compliant patient, the rehabilitation program will not be successful. To ensure compliance, it is important to inform the patient of the content of the program and the expected course of rehabilitation.

- I: Individualization. Each person responds differently to an injury and to the subsequent rehabilitation program. Even though an injury may seem the same in type and severity as another, undetectable differences can change an individual's response to it. Individual physiological and chemical differences profoundly affect a patient's specific responses to an injury.

- S: Specific sequencing. A therapeutic exercise program should follow a specific sequence of events. This specific sequence is determined by the body's physiological healing response.

- I: Intensity. The intensity level of the therapeutic exercise program must challenge the patient and the injured area but at the same time must not cause aggravation. Knowing when to increase intensity without overtaxing the injury requires observation of the patient's response and consideration of the healing process.

- T: Total patient. It must be considered the total patient in the rehabilitation process. It is important for the unaffected areas of the body to stay finely tuned. This means keeping the cardiovascular system at a preinjury level and maintaining range of motion, strength, coordination, and muscle endurance of the uninjured limbs and joints. The whole body must be the focus of the rehabilitation program, not just the injured area. Providing the patient with a program to keep the uninvolved areas in peak condition, rather than just rehabilitating the injured area, will help to better prepare the patient physically and psychologically for when the injured area is completely rehabilitated.

Components

Regardless of the specifics of the injury, however, here are fundamental components that need to be included in all successful rehabilitation programs:

Pain Management

Medications are a mainstay of treatment in the injured athlete - both for their pain relief and healing properties. It is recommended that they need to be used judiciously with a distinct regard for the risks and side effects as well as the potential benefits, which include pain relief and early return to play. Therapeutic modalities play a small, but important, part in the rehabilitation of sports injuries. They may help to decrease pain and edema to allow an exercise-based rehabilitation programme to proceed. By understanding the physiological basis of these modalities, a safe and appropriate treatment choice can be made, but its effectiveness will ultimately depend upon the patient's individualized and subjective response to treatment.

Flexibility and Joint ROM

Injury or surgery can result in decreased joint ROM mainly due to fibrosis and wound contraction. Besides that, it is common for post-injury flexibility to be diminished as a result of muscle spasm, inflammation, swelling and pain. In addition to impacting the injured area, this also affects the joints above and below the problem, and creates motor pattern issues. Flexibility training is an important component of rehabilitation in order to minimize the decrease in joint ROM. Also, a variety of stretching techniques can be used in improving range of motion, including PNF, ballistic stretching and static stretching.

Strength and Endurance

Injuries to the musculoskeletal system could result in skeletal muscle hypotrophy and weakness, loss of aerobic capacity and fatigability. During rehabilitation after a sports injury it is important to try to maintain cardiovascular endurance. Thus regular bicycling, one-legged bicycling or arm cycling, an exercise programme in a pool using a wet vest or general major muscle exercise programmes with relatively high intensity and short rest periods (circuit weight training) can be of major importance.

Proprioception and Coordination

Proprioception can be defined as 'a special type of sensitivity that informs about the sensations of the deep organs and of the relationship between muscles and joints'. Loss of proprioception occurs with injury to ligaments, tendons, or joints, and also with immobilization. Proprioceptive re-education has to get the muscular receptors working, in order to provide a rapid motor response. Restoration of proprioception is an important part of rehabilitation. The treatment has to be adapted to each individual, considering the type of injury and the stress to which the athlete will be exposed when practicing his or her sport.

Coordination can be defined as 'the capacity to perform movements in a smooth, precise and controlled manner'. Rehabilitation techniques increasingly refer to neuromuscular re-education. Improving coordination depends on repeating the positions and movements associated with different sports and correct training. It has to begin with simple activities, performed slowly and perfectly executed, gradually increasing in speed and complexity. The technician should make sure that the athlete performs these movements unconsciously, until they finally become automatic.

Functional Rehabilitation

All rehabilitation programs must take into account, and reproduce, the activities and movements required when the athlete returns to the field post-injury. The goal of function-based rehabilitation programmes is the return of the athlete to optimum athletic function. Optimal athletic function is the result of physiological motor activations creating specific biomechanical motions and positions using intact anatomical structures to generate forces and actions.

Use of Orthotics

The use of orthotic devices to support musculoskeletal function and the correction of muscle imbalances and inflexibility in uninjured areas should receive the attention of the rehabilitation team. Appropriate orthotic application will result in restraint forces that oppose an undesired motion. A complete orthotic prescription should include the patient's diagnosis, consider the type of footwear to be used, include the joints it encompasses and specify the desired biomechanical alignment, as well as the materials for fabrication. Communication with the orthotist,who will fabricate or fit the brace, is of utmost importance in order to obtain a good clinical result.

Psychology of Injury

Injury is more than physical; that is, the athlete must be psychologically ready for the demands of his or her sport. The most immediate emotional response at the point of injury is shock. It's degree may range from minor to significant, depending upon the severity of the injury. It is important to note that denial itself is an adaptive response that allows an individual to manage extreme emotional responses to situational stress. Many individuals assist athletes through the recovery process and can foster psychological readiness, but they can also identify those who are physically recovered but require more time or intervention to be fully prepared to return to competition. Thus, rehabilitation and recovery are not purely physical but also psychological.

Mental skills in sports are often viewed as part of an individual's personality and something that cannot be taught. Many physicians feel that injured athletes either have or do not have the mental toughness to progress through rehabilitation. Mental skills, however, can be learned. One example for this is to provide proper goal setting, which has very important role in sports rehabilitation, because they can enhance recovery from injury. Goal setting needs to be measurable and stated in behavioral terms. The research indicates that goals should be challenging and difficult, yet attainable. It is important for physicians to help them focus on short-term goals as a means to attain long-term goals. For example, to set daily and weekly goals in rehabilitation process which will end in long-term goal like returning to play after an injury. It is important for sports medicine physicians to assist patients in setting goals related to performance process rather than outcomes, such as returning to play.

Stages of Rehabilitation

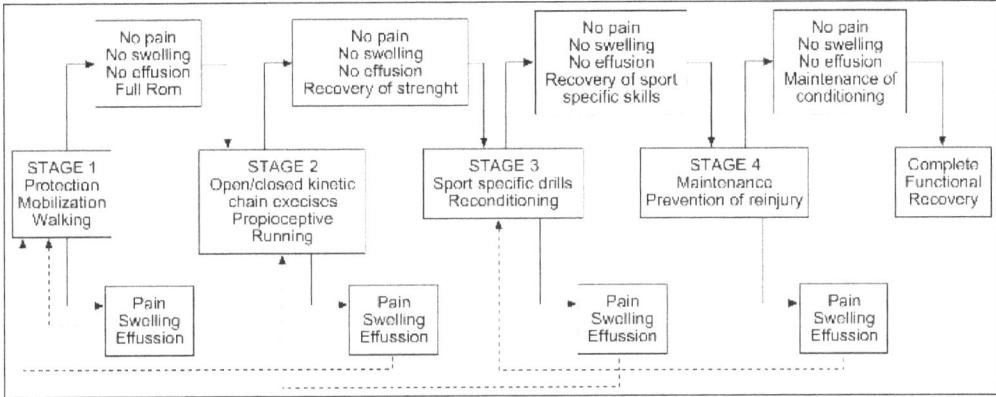

Initial Stage of Rehabilitation

This phase lasts approximately 4-6 days. The body's first response to an injury is inflammation. It's main function is to defend the body against harmful substances, dispose of dead or dying tissue and to promote the renewal of normal tissue. The goals during the initial phase of the rehabilitation process include limitation of tissue damage, pain relief, control of the inflammatory response to injury, and protection of the affected anatomical area. The pathological events that take place immediately after the injury could lead to impairments such as muscle atrophy and weakness and limitation in the joint range of motion. These impairments result in functional losses, for example, inability to jump or lift an object. The extent of the functional loss may be influenced by the nature and timing of the therapeutic and rehabilitative intervention during the initial phase of the injury. If functional losses are severe or become permanent, the athlete now with a disability may be unable to participate in his/her sport.

The physiotherapist is usually the professional in charge of this phase although the process may be started by a medical doctor.

Control Pain and Swelling

Primary treatment in initial phase of rehabilitation is RICE. It is the term that stands for Rest, Ice, Compression and Elevation. RICE can be used immediately and 24 to 48 hours after many muscle strains, ligament sprains, or other bruises and injuries.

Therapeutic modalities and medications are used to create an optimal environment for injury repair by limiting the inflammatory process and breaking the pain-spasm cycle. Use of any modality depends on the supervising physician's exercise prescription, as well as the injury site, and type and severity of injury. In some cases, a modality may be indicated and contraindicated for the same condition. For example, thermotherapy (heat therapy) may be contraindicated for tendinitis during the initial phase of the exercise program. However, once acute inflammation is controlled, heat therapy may be indicated. Frequent evaluation of the individual's progress is necessary to ensure that the appropriate modality is being used.

Despite the fact that rapid return to competition is crucial, rest is necessary to protect the damaged tissue from additional injury. Therefore, exercise involving the injured area is not recomended during this phase, although there are a few exceptions such as the tendinopathy protocols used to rehabilitate Achilles and patella tendon injuries. However, it is important to realize that a quick return to function relies on the health of other body tissues.

The power, strength, and endurance of the musculoskeletal tissues and the function of the cardiorespiratory system must be maintained. Athlete needs to understands the reasons for following a particular treatment regime or exercise program, as well medical professional's advice should be sought before embarking on any regime as more harm can be done than good if carried out incorrectly.

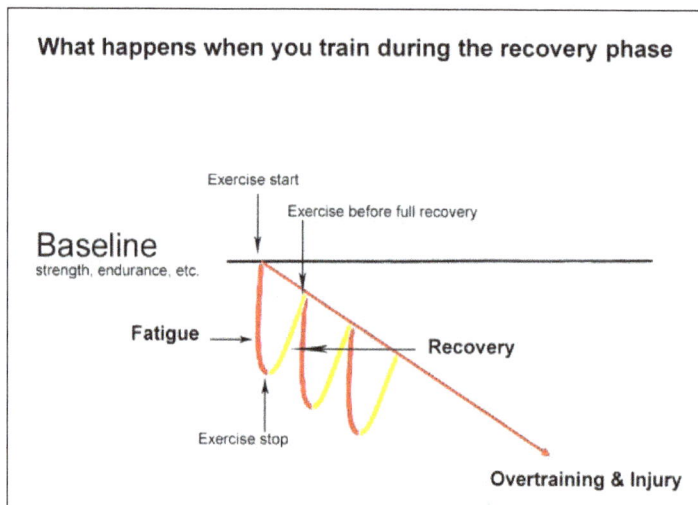

What happens when you train during the recovery phase

Exercise start

Exercise before full recovery

Baseline
strength, endurance, etc.

Fatigue ⟶

⟵ Recovery

Exercise stop

Overtraining & Injury

Active range of motion is performed under one's own control, while passive range of motion occurs when another person or device produces the movement. If movement of the injured limb is not contraindicated, isolated exercises that target areas proximal and distal to the injured area may be permissible provided that they do not stress the injured area. Examples include hip abduction and rotation exercises following knee injury or scapula stabilizing exercises following glenohumeral joint injury. Isometric exercises are used for strengthening when range of motion is restricted or needs to be avoided due to the fracture or acute inflammation of a joint. Otherwise, isotonic strengthening can begin within the painless arc of joint motion.

Intermediate Stage of Rehabilitation

This phase lasts from day 5 to 8-10 weeks. After the inflammatory phase, the body begins to repair the damaged tissue with similar tissue, but the resiliency of the new tissue is low. Repair of the weakened injury site can take up to eight weeks if the proper amount of restorative stress is applied, or longer if too much or too little stress is applied.

Joint ROM and Muscle Conditioning

The goals during the second phase of rehabilitation include the limitation of the impairment and the recovery from the functional losses. Early protected motion hastens the optimal alignment of collagen fibers and promotes improved tissue mobility. A number of physical modalities are used to enhance tissue healing. Exercise to regain flexibility, strength, endurance, balance, and coordination become the central component of the intervention. To the extent that these impairments and functional losses were minimized by early intervention, progress in this phase can be accelerated. Again, the maintenance of muscular and cardiorespiratory function remains essential for the uninjured areas of the body. The strength and conditioning professional has considerable expertise to offer the other members of the sports medicine team regarding selection of the appropriate activities.

Possible exercise forms during this phase include strengthening of the uninjured extremities and areas proximal and distal to the injury, aerobic and anaerobic exercise, and improving strength and neuromuscular control of the involved areas:

- Isometric exercise may be performed provided that it is pain free and otherwise indicated. Submaximal isometric exercise allows the athlete to maintain neuromuscular function and improve strength with movements performed at an intensity low enough that the newly formed collagen fibers are not disrupted.

- Isokinetic exercise can be an important aspect of strengthening following injury. This type of exercise uses equipment that provides resistance to movement at a given speed (e.g., 60°/s or 120°/s). Isotonic exercise involves movements with constant external resistance and the amount of force required to move the resistance varies, depending primarily on joint angle and the length of each agonist muscle. Isotonic exercise uses several different forms of resistance, including gravity (i.e., exercises performed without equipment, with gravitational effects as the only source of resistance), dumbbells, barbells, and weight-stack machines. The speed at which the movement occurs is controlled by the athlete; movement speed can be a program design variable, with more acute injuries calling for slower movement and the later phases of healing amenable to faster, more sport-specific movement.

- Specific types of exercises exist to improve neuromuscular control following injury and can be manipulated through alterations in surface stability, vision, and speed. Mini-trampolines, balance boards, and stability balls can be used to create unstable surfaces for upper and lower extremity training. Athletes can perform common activities such as squats and push-ups on uneven surfaces to improve neuromuscular control.

- Exercises may also be performed with eyes closed, thus removing visual input, to further challenge balance.

Finally, increasing the speed at which exercises are performed provides additional challenges to the system. Specifically controlling these variables within a controlled environment will allow the athlete to progress to more challenging exercises in the next stage of healing.

Advanced Stage of Rehabilitation

This phase begins at around 21 days and can continue for 6-12 months. The outcome of the previous phase is the replacement of damaged tissue with collagen fibers. After those fibers are laid down, the body can begin to remodel and strengthen the new tissue, allowing the athlete to gradually return to full activity. This phase of rehabilitation represents the start of the conditioning process needed to return to sports training and competition. Understanding the demands of the particular sport becomes essential as well as communication with the coach. This phase also represents an opportunity to identify and correct risk factors, thus reducing the possibility of re-injury.

Functional Training

The combination of clinic-based and sport-specific functional techniques will provide an individualized, sport-specific rehabilitation protocol for the athlete. Rehabilitation and reconditioning exercises must be functional to facilitate a return to competition. Examples of functional training include joint angle-specific strengthening, velocity-specific muscle activity, closed kinetic chain exercises, and exercises designed to further enhance neuromuscular control. Strengthening should transition from general exercises to sport-specific exercises designed to replicate movements common in given sports. Cross-training is encouraged, especially with activities that do not produce any symptoms from the injury.

It is essential that the rehabilitation and training be sufficiently vigorous to prepare the injured tissue for the demands of the game. With each increase in activity, signs of recurring pain or weakness should trigger a slowdown or a reversal to a tolerable level of activity. The player will have returned to game during this phase and will have ceased physiotherapy or individual rehabilitation while this process is still continuing. Unrestricted sports activity is not allowed until all of these steps have been completed and full-effort sports-specific activity is tolerated without symptoms.

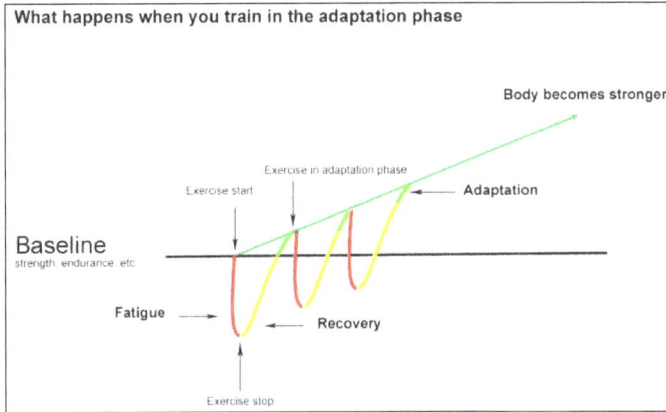

Return to Sport

At some point in the recovery process, athletes return to strength and conditioning programs and resume sport-specific activities in preparation for return to play. The transition is important for several reasons. First, although the athlete may have recovered in medical terms (ie, improvements in flexibility, range of motion, functional strength, pain, neuromuscular control, inflammation), preparation for competition requires the restoration of strength, power, speed, agility, and endurance at levels exhibited in sport.

Return to play is defined as the process of deciding when an injured or ill athlete may safely return to practice or competition. Early return to training and sport are considered sensible goals if the rate of return is based on the affected muscle, the severity of the injury and the position of the athlete.

Criteria for return to play must emphasize gradual return to sport-specific functional progressions. Sport-specific function occurs when the activations, motions and resultant forces are specific and efficient for the needs of that sport. Sport-specific functional rehabilitation should focus on restoration of the injured athlete's ability to have sport-specific physiology and biomechanics to interact optimally with the sport-specific demands. That means that they need to be replicated at the same speed, on the same surface and with the same level of fatigue to be truly effective.

Once a athlete has been medically cleared to return-to-play there are some fundamental steps that need to be followed:

- The athlete has to fulfill the fitness standards of the team he is returning to.

- The athlete needs to pass some skill specific tests applicable to his playing position.

- The player may then begin practicing with the team.

- Exposure to the match situation should be gradual, with the match time gradually increasing.

There are simple guidelines which need to be developed by each team with contributions and support from each member of the medical team.

Monitoring

Regarding these aspects from the text above, there are several problems: are all the mechanic parameters of the performance (force, velocity, power) regained at that time? Are there any ways to conduct the rehabilitation program in order to obtain better parameters and so the return to the sports activity to be safely done? Which could be the most suitable evaluation methods in order to be sure about the athletes well-training?

Monitoring athlete well-being is essential to guide training and to detect any progression towards negative health outcomes and associated poor performance. Objective (performance, physiological, biochemical) and subjective measures (mood disturbance, perceived stress and recovery and symptoms of stress) are all options for athlete monitoring. Appropriate load monitoring can aid in determining whether an athlete is adapting to a training program and in minimizing the risk of developing non-functional overreaching, illness, and/or injury.

In order to gain an understanding of the training load and its effect on the athlete, a number of potential markers are available for use. There are a number of external load quantifying and monitoring tools, such as power output measuring devices, time-motion analysis, as well as internal load unit measures, including perception of effort, heart rate, blood lactate, and training impulse. Other monitoring tools used by high-performance programs include heart rate recovery, neuromuscular function, biochemical/hormonal/immunological assessments, questionnaires and diaries, psychomotor speed, and sleep quality and quantity. Coaching staffs and administrative personnel must work to ensure that care can be provided at all points of the rehabilitation process, especially when funding dictates the need to hire personnel capable of addressing injuries at multiple levels. A clear understanding of the injury and of the interventions from each provider is vital to an efficient and successful return to play.

Appropriate monitoring of training load can provide important information to athletes and coaches; however, monitoring systems should be intuitive, provide efficient data analysis and interpretation, and enable efficient reporting of simple, yet scientifically valid, feedback. If accurate and easy-to-interpret feedback is provided to the athlete and coach, load monitoring can result in enhanced knowledge of training responses, aid in the design of training programs, provide a further avenue for communication between support staff and athletes and coaches and ultimately enhance an athlete's performance.

Benefits of Sport Specific Rehabilitation

For the discerning athlete, there is simply no comparison between general rehabilitation after an injury and rehabilitation after a sports-related injury. For one, their goals are different. Sport specific rehab goes beyond recovery. It focuses on the mechanics and forces of your sport to prepare you to play again with equal or even better performance than before.

When your body is used to the rigors of athletic activities, basic rehab just isn't enough. You need an experienced sports physical therapist to get you back into prime condition to return to the sport you love.

Sports injuries are incredibly common as more people seek healthier lifestyles and encourage their children to participate in youth sports. One study finds 8.6 million Americans suffered a sports-related injury in one year. Many of these injuries can be treated at home while others require some hospitalization. If you are hospitalized for a sports injury, you will likely require physical therapy, too.

Physical therapy is necessary for a full recovery after a sports-related injury. Often injured body parts must be immobilized or rested while they heal. During the healing process, those muscles and joints get out of practice, so to speak. As part of rehabilitation process, you need to exercise the injured area to build up strength and regain normal function. Physical therapy teaches you how to do this safely so you regain mobility efficiently and avoid further injury.

Sports physical therapy for athletes is especially important. Whereas regular physical therapy helps patients recover the ability to perform daily living activities, sports physical therapy restores your body's ability to withstand the extreme stress of athletics.

Sports PT targets the specific needs of your sport. Every sport requires different movements and mechanics and exerts different forces on your body. Where a weightlifter needs more focus on strength and conditioning, a runner will benefit more from gait analysis. A sports physical therapist can give you tailored exercises to address the specific strain of your sport and prepare you to perform under those stresses again.

Sports PT also considers your unique body composition that can affect your athletic performance as well as your rehabilitation. Your sports physical therapist can recognize how your body works and help you correct pre-existing physiological imbalances or potentially damaging patterns of motion that put you at risk for further injury.

Sport specific rehabilitation is the best course of action to restore and enhance your original athletic abilities when you have suffered a debilitating sports injury. There are many other benefits to sports PT that will aid in your recovery, such as:

- Pain management.

- Increased cellular metabolism to encourage healing of damaged tissue.

- Increased circulation in the injured area to encouraging healing.

- Strengthening of weakened muscles.

- Prevention of muscular atrophy.

- Stimulation of joint receptors.

- Restoration of range of motion and increased flexibility in tight muscles.

- Increased lymphatic drainage.

- Increased extensibility of connective and supporting tissue structures.

- Relief of muscular spasms.

Ultimately, sport specific rehab is designed to help you heal faster and more completely while minimizing pain and preventing further injury. Don't just settle for general rehabilitation. With proper sports PT, athletes of all skill levels can return to their sport better than ever.

Ankle and Foot Injuries in Athletes

The foot and ankle are among the most common sites for both acute and chronic injuries in athletes and other physically active individuals.[1] Although seldom life-threatening, they often have detrimental effects on sport activity and participation. When an injury to the foot or ankle occurs athletes are limited in their abilities to run, jump, kick, and change directions. Thus, the treatment and rehabilitation of these injuries are crucial in returning athletes to full participation at full functioning. When managing injuries for the foot and ankle, all of the typical clinical considerations must be thought of (type of injury, severity, healing time, type and level of activity, etc), but it is also important to consider other factors such as foot type, biomechanics, footwear worn during activity, and external supports such as bracing or taping. The foot is the base of the lower quarter kinetic chain, thus if rehabilitation and treatment is not managed properly, an injury to the foot or ankle can ultimately cause secondary injuries elsewhere up the chain.

Biomechanics of Normal Walking

For all sports medicine specialists, evaluation of gait is important for the rehabilitation of lower extremity injuries. Understanding the normal gait pattern will enable a clinician to identify and correct improper compensations after injury. The identification of gait abnormalities should play a key component in deciding to refer a patient for supervised rehabilitation. The movement of the lower extremity during normal walking and running can be divided into two phases, the stance phase and the swing phase.

The stance or support phase, starts with initial contact at heel strike and ends at toe-off. This phase has two important functions. First, at heel strike, the foot acts like a shock absorber to the impact forces and then the foot adapts to the surface. Secondly, at toe-off the foot functions as a rigid level to transmit the force from the foot to the surface. At initial contact, the subtalar joint is supinated and there is an external rotation of the tibia. As the foot loads, the subtalar joint moves into a pronated position until the fore-foot is in contact with the ground. The change in subtalar motion occurs between initial heel strike and 20 percent into the support phase of running. As pronation occurs at the subtalar joint the tibia will rotate internally. Transverse plane rotation occurs at the knee joint because of this tibial rotation. Pronation of the foot unlocks the midtarsal joint and allows the foot to assist in shock absorption and to adapt to the uneven surfaces. It is important during initial impact to reduce the ground reaction forces and to distribute the load evenly on many different anatomical structures throughout the foot and leg. Pronation is normal and allows for this distribution of forces on as many structures as possible to avoid excessive loading on just a few structures. The subtalar joint remains in a pronated position until 55 to 85 percent of the support phase with maximam pronation is concurrent with the body's center of gravity passing over the base of support. From 70 to 90 percent of the support phase, the foot begins to resupinate and will approach the neutral subtalar position. In supination the midtarsal joints are locked and the foot be-comes stable and rigid to prepare for push-off. This rigid position allows the foot to exert a greater amount of force from the lower extremity to the surface. The swing phase begins immediately after toe-off and ends as just prior to heel-strike. During the swing phase the leg is moved from behind the body to a position in front of the body.

Lateral Ankle Sprain

Lateral ankle sprains are common acute injuries suffered by athletes. The most common mechanism for a lateral ankle sprain is excessive inversion and plantar flexion of the rea-foot on the tibia. The injured ligaments are located on the lateral aspect of the ankle and include the anterior talofibular, the posterior talofibular, and the calcaneofibular.

With lateral ankle sprains, the severity of the ligament damage will determine the classi-fication and course of treatment. In a grade 1 sprain, there is stretching of the ligaments with little or no joint instability. Pain and swelling for a grade 1 sprain are often mild and seldom debilitating. After initial management for pain and swelling of the grade 1 sprain, rehabilitation can often be started immediately. Time loss from physical activity for a grade 1 sprain is typically less than one week. Grade 2 sprains occur with some tearing of ligamentous fibers and moderate instability of the joint. Pain and swelling are moderate to severe and often immobilization is required for several days. With a grade 3 sprain, there is total rupture of the ligament with gross instability of the joint. Pain and swelling is so debilitating that weight bearing is impossible for up to several weeks.

Rehabilitation Expectations

With lateral ankle sprains regaining full range of motion, strength, and neuromuscular coordination are paramount during rehabilitation. Isometrics and open-chain range of motion can be completed by those patients who are non-weight bearing. Range of motion should focus on dorsiflexion and plantar flexion and be performed passively and actively as tolerated. During early rehabilitation, towel stretches, and wobble board range of motion should be introduced as tolerated. Stationary biking can aid dorsiflexion and plantar flexion motion in a controlled environment while also providing a cardiovascular workout for the athlete. Clinicians can also incorporate joint mobilizations to aid in dorsiflexion range of motion. Hydrotherapy is an excellent means to work on range of motion while also gaining the benefits of hydrostatic pressure.

Once weight bearing is tolerated, middle stage rehabilitation is started. This includes balance and neuromuscular control exercises as well as continued range of motion exercises as tolerated. Balance activities should progress from double-limbed stance to single-limb stance as well as from a firm surface to progressively more unstable surfaces. Closing the eyes or incorporating perturbations can further challenge patients. Patients can be asked to throw and catch weighted balls, perform single leg squats, and perform single limb balance and reaching exercises. Regaining and maintaining range of motion should be continued. Wobble board training and slant board stretches are also important to focus on heel cord stretching.

A

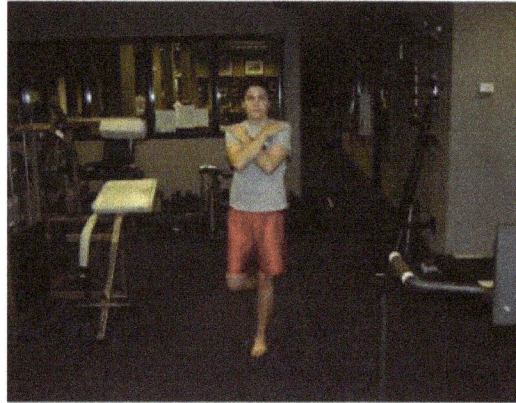

B

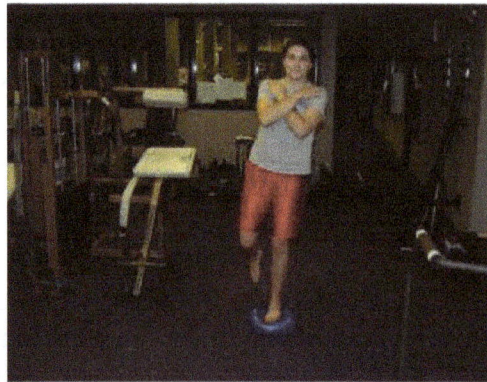

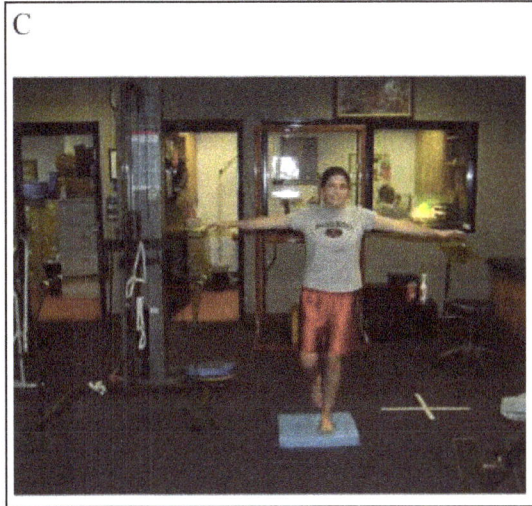

Balance training exercises include single limb standing. These exercises can be progressed by changing arm position, closing the eyes, and adding an unstable surface under the foot.

Increased strengthening exercises should be started once swelling and pain is controlled. Initially, dorsiflexion and plantar flexion strength should be focused on. Weight bearing calf raises and squats are examples excellent beginning exercises. As the ligaments heal, inversion and eversion strengthening should be added as tolerated. Resistance bands and ankle weights are a good means to gain strength in all planes of motion. Clinicians can integrate diagonal exercises (i.e, combined plantar flexion/inversion and dorsiflexion/eversion) to isolate motions at the talocrural joint.

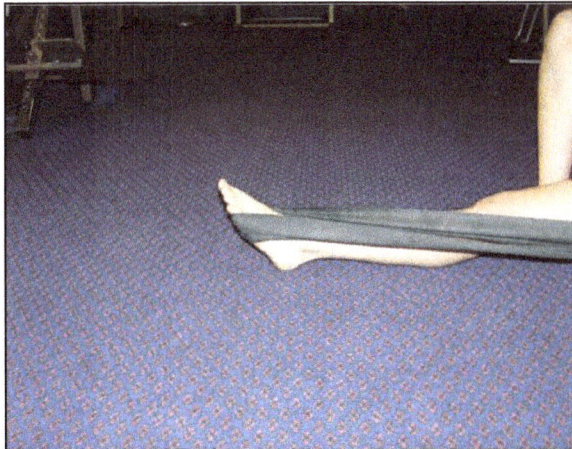

Strength training may be performed with resistance tubing exercises.

During this time, it is paramount for clinicians to re-educate athletes on the proper mechanics of walking. Once range of motion and strength is regained, functional activities are included. Functional rehabilitation exercises should begin with simple, uniplaner exercises; walking and jogging in a straight line. Once the athlete can perform these without a pain or a limp, hops, jumps, skips and change of direction can start to be added. Have the athlete perform 10 jumps for distance on the uninvolved limb and challenge him/her to match the distance with the involved limb. Do the same for jumps for height. As cutting is started, begin with wide arching turns and progress to tighter, sharper and faster cuts. Athletes should be challenged to perform lateral movements as well such as shuffling and carioca. As the patient becomes more comfortable and functional, have him/her perform rehab wearing the typical shoe/cleat for the sport and progress to more sport specific activities.

Depending on the severity of the ankle sprain, fear avoidance may cause the athlete to alter play and be at higher risk for reinjury or injury to another location. Also, some sport-specific skills may need to be reconditioned. Participation into sport should start with non-contact drills and progress to contact drills and finally to full scrimmage.

Criteria for Full Competition

Full return to activity should be a gradual progression in order to stress the ligaments without causing further harm. Full activity should be allowed once the athlete has complete range of motion, 80 to 90 percent of preinjury strength, and a normal gait pattern including the ability to perform sport-specific tasks such as cutting and landing without any compensations due to the injury. The athlete should be capable, without pain or swelling to complete a full practice.

Clinical Pearls

- Challenge patients with home-exercises. Have them try to balance on involved limb while brushing teeth, progress to eyes shut while brushing their teeth and balancing.

- Have rehabilitation clinicians perform talocrural and tibiofibular joint mobilizations to increase dorsiflexion.

- Perform exercises with shoes on and off to alter the planter cutaneous feedback.

- Using a 10-20 yard area, have the patient walk on toes back in forth. Repeat walking with toes pointed in, toes pointed out, and on heels (toes in the air).

- Ask the subject to perform 10 single leg jumps in a row on the involved limb as high as possible in a row, while watching his/her face, if he/she can complete without grimacing safe to start functional rehabilitation.

Patient Education

The leading predisposing factor for an ankle sprain is a history of an ankle sprain and an estimated 30% of all individuals who suffer an initial ankle sprain will develop chronic ankle instability. Thus, patients need to know that inadequate treatment and rehabilitation of an ankle sprain has a great likelihood of leading to future problems.

Often patients, coaches, and parents have the mindset that a lateral ankle sprain is not serious and players can return quickly. In fact, in many cases health care services are not even sought by individuals suffering an ankle sprain It is critical for all stakeholders to understand the high frequency of residual symptoms and recurrent sprains. The importance of allowing the ligaments to heal, regaining full range of motion, strength, and balance prior to returning to activity must be emphasized to patients. If, while doing rehabilitation swelling returns, patients must know that they did too much.

Prophylactic Support

Prophylactic support is often used after an ankle sprain to provide mechanical stability. Depending upon individual preference and budget, athletes can use tape or a variety of braces (lace-up, stirrup, or elastic type of configuration. Both taping and bracing have been found to reduce the risk of recurrent ankle sprains in athletes. Advantages of a braces include easy of application and cost effectiveness. Braces also provide the athlete with proprioceptive stimulation, which implies an improve proprioception and sensory feedback. Taping, one the other hand can be custom designed for the specific athlete, sport, and instabilities.

Other Ankle Sprains

Although less common, medial and syndesmodic ankle sprains often result in more severe injuries causing longer time to heal and rehabilitate. Medial ankle sprains occur with a mechanism of excessive eversion and dorsiflexion, causing the deltoid ligament to be injured. Patients with medial ankle sprains will often present with swelling and discoloration on the medial aspect of the ankle and unwillingness to bear weight.

Syndesmodic sprains occur with disruption of the interosseous (or syndesmodic) ligament that stabilizing the inferior tibiofibular joint. Injury to this ligament occurs with excessive external rotational or forced dorsiflexion. Syndesmotic sprains may occur in isolation or in combination with medial or lateral ankle sprains. Due to limited blood supply and the difficulty in allowing the injured ligament to heal unless the ankle is immobilized, injuries to the syndesmodic ligaments often take months to heal. Patients with syndesmodic sprains often present with a lack of swelling, but will be extremely tender over anterior aspect of the distal tibiofibular joint.

Rehabilitation Expectations

Initial treatment for both medial and syndesmodic sprains is often immobilization and crutches. During this time, swelling and pain management are the primary concerns. The length of time of immobilization will vary among patients and will depend on the severity of the sprain. While immobilized, patients can work on controlled open-chain range of motion, focusing on dorsiflexion and plantar flexion. During this time, inversion and eversion should be held to a minimum. During early rehabilitation, nothing should increase pain or swelling to the area.

Once weight-bearing is tolerated, crutches should be used at a minimum. Gait training may be needed to ensure the patient is not compensating in any way, which may cause secondary injury. At this point, rehabilitation will follow the progression as stated above in the lateral ankle section. Rehabilitation concerns include; pain and swelling, range of motion, strength, balance and neuromuscular control, and functional exercises.

Criteria for Full Competition

Full return to activity should be a gradual progression in order to stress the ligaments without causing further harm. Full activity should be allowed once the athlete has complete range of motion, 80 to 90 percent of preinjury strength, and the ability to perform gait activities (including running and changing direction) without difficulty.. The athlete should be capable, without pain or swelling to complete a full practice.

Patient Education

With medial and syndesmodic sprains, patience is the most important thing for the patient to learn. The healing of the medial and syndesmodic ligaments take time, sometimes up to severalmonths to fully heal. The difference in the expectations of these injuries compared to lateral ankle sprains must be emphasized to all stakeholders so that realistic expectations for return to play can be understood.

Plantar Fasciitis

Plantar fasciitis is the catchall term that is commonly used to describe pain on the plantar aspect of the proximal arch and heel. The plantar fascia is an aporneurosis that runs the length of the sole of the foot and is a broad dense band of connective tissue. It is attached proximally to the medial surface of the calcaneus and fans out distally, attaching to the metatarsophalangeal articulations and merges into the capsular ligaments. The plantar aponeurosis assists in maintaining the stability of the foot and secures or braces the longitudinal arch.

Plantar fasciitis is caused by a straining of the fascia near its origin. The plantar fascia is under tension with toe extension and depression of the longitudinal arch. During normal standing (weight bearing principally on the heel), the fascia is under minimal stress, however, when the weight is shifted to the balls of the feet (running) the fascia is put under stress and strain. Often planar fasciitis is a result of chronic running with poor technique, poor footwear, or because of lordosis, a condition in which the increased forward tilt of the pelvis produces an unfavorable angle of foot-strike when there is considerable force exerted on the ball of the foot.

Patients more prone to plantar fasciitis include: those with a pes cavus foot; excessive pronation; overweight; walking, running or standing for long periods of time, especially on hard surfaces; old, worn shoes (insufficient arch support); and tight Achilles tendon. The patient will present with pain in the anterior medial heel, usually at the attachment of the plantar fascia to the calcaneus. The pain is particularly noticeable during the first couple of steps in the morning or after sitting for a long time. Often the pain will lessen as the patient moves more, however the pain will increase if the athlete is on his/her feet excessively or on his/her toes often. Upon inspection, the plantar fascia may or may not be swollen with crepitus. The patient's pain will increase with forefoot and toe dorsiflexion.

Rehabilitation Expectations

Depending on patient compliance, plantar fasciitis can be a very treatable minor injury with symptoms lasting days. However, without proper treatment and patient compliance, plantar fasciitis can linger for months or even years.

Initial treatment of plantar fasciitis starts with pain control. Rest is extremely important at this time, patients should not being performing any unnecessary weight bearing. Patients should also be wearing comfortable supportive shoes when walking is necessary. Adding a heel cup or custom foot orthosis to a patient's shoe may relieve some of the pain at the plantar fascia insertion. During this time, regaining full dorsiflexion range of motion of the foot as well as of the big toe is vital. Towel stretches, slant board stretches, and joint mobilizations administered by a rehabilitation clinician will aid in the return of dorsiflexion range of motion.

After pain is reduced strengthening exercises can be incorporated into rehabilitatoin. The focus should be in strengthening some of the smaller extrinsic and intrinsic muscles of the foot. Towel crutches, big toe-little toes raises, short foot exercises are good examples of strengthening exercises. Throughout the treatment and rehabilitation process, soft tissue work such as cross-friction massage may aid in the alleviation of symptoms.

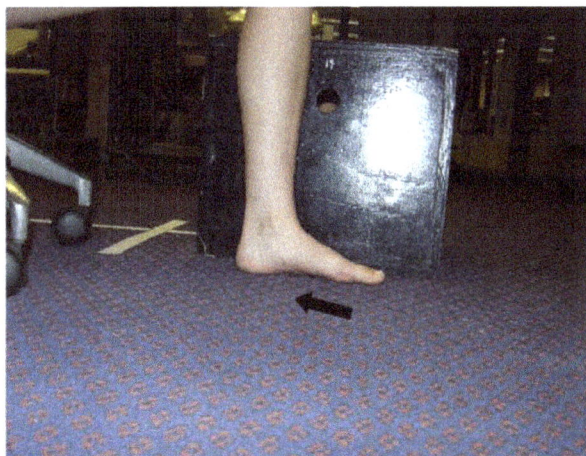

Short foot exercises are performed by contracting the plantar intrinsic muscles in an effort
to pull the metatarsal heads towards the calcaneus. Emphasis should
be placed on minimizing extrinsic muscle activity.

Criteria for Full Competition

Although athletes can often continue to participate fully while suffering from plantar fasciitis, it should be understood that the longer activity is continued, the longer the symptoms will linger. For best recovery of this injury, extra activity should not be started until the athlete is able to walk a full day without any pain. Once a daily activities are tolerated, activity can slowly be increased until full participation. Throughout the rehabilitation and participation progression stretching should occur often throughout the day.

Clinical Pearls

- While sitting, roll on a ball (tennis ball, golf ball, etc) underneath the medial longitudinal to stretch the plantar fascia.

- Fill a paper cup with water and freeze it, roll on the frozen cup to get the benefits of cold while also stretching the plantar fascia.

- Before getting out of bed in the morning, but on shoes with good arch supports to provide the plantar fascia support upon weight-bearing.

- Sleep with feet off the end of the bed to allow some dorsiflexion while sleeping.

- Wear a night splint that will keep foot in a dorsiflexed or neutral position.

- Stretching often throughout the day for a short period of time is more beneficial then stretching once a day for a long period of time.

- Do not weight high-heels or other shoes with no support (sandals) during the day.

Patient Education

Plantar fascia tends to be a cyclical injury. Athletes will repetitively suffer from this injury because after the initial injury, the cause of the injury is not treated, only the symptoms. Patients with plantar fasciitis need to have their gait biomechanics thoroughly evaluated and, if necessary, be fitted for custom orthotics.

Achilles Tendonitis

Achilles tendonitis is an inflammatory condition that involves the Achilles tendon and/or its tendon sheath. Achilles tendonitis is the most common overuse injuries reported in distance runners. Although Achilles tendonitis is generally a chronic condition, acute injury may also occur. Typically, the athlete will suffer from gradual pain and stiffness about the Achilles tendon region, 2 to 6 cm proximal to the calcaneal insertion. The pain will increase after running hills, stairs, or an increased amount of sprints (running on toes). Upon evaluation, the gastrocnemius and soleus muscle testing may be normal however, flexibility will be reduced. Having the patient perform toe raises to fatigue will show a deficit compared to the uninvolved limb. Inspection of the area may feel warm to the touch and pain, tenderness and crepitus may be felt with palpation. The tendon may appear thickened indicating a chronic condition.

Rehabilitation Expectations

Healing of Achilles tendonitis is a slow process due to the lack of vascularity to the tendon. Initially, patients will feel comfortable by placing less stress to the area by wearing a heel cup. Resting and activity modification is important during the initially healing stages. The clinician needs to emphasize the importance of allowing the tendon to heal. During this time, cross friction massage can be started to the area to break down adhesions and promote blood flow to the area.

Stretching and strengthening of the gastrocnemious-soleus complex should be incorporated as tolerated by the patient. Towel stretching and slant board stretching should be done throughout the day. As range of motion is restored, the heel cup should be removed to reduce the chances of adaptive shortening of the muscles and tendon. Progressive strengthening including toe raises and resistive tubing should be incorporated at the beginning of rehabilitation. Sets should start low with low reps and gradually increase to low sets high reps for endurance as tolerated by the athlete. As pain and inflammation decreases, machine weights, lunges, and sport specific exercises can be added. Eccentric exercises for the triceps surae often have beneficial results in athletes with Achilles tendonitis.

The patient's foot structure and gait mechanics should be evaluated for possible orthotic benefits. Often Achilles tendonitis is a result of overpronation, an abnormality that can be addressed with foot orthoses. Once range of motion, strength and endurance has returned, athletes should slowly progress into walking and jogging program. Workouts should be done on a flat surface when possible. The walking and jogging program should start out with slow mini-bursts of speed. The program is to increase the amount of stress the Achilles tendon can tolerate; it is not to improve overall endurance. As tolerated by the patient, running and sprinting can be increased.

Criteria for Full Competition

Athletes should be allowed to compete when full range of motion and strength has returned. The athlete should have regained endurance in the involved limb and be capable of completing a full practice without pain. Depending on the sport, some athletes may be able to compete while suffering from Achilles tendonitis. However, patients should be educated in the fact that the condition will not go away without proper rest and treatment.

Patient Education

Patients need to be educated with the risks of Achilles tendonitis, specifically hill running, lack of proper shoes, lack of rest, and flexibility. Hill workouts increase the stress and strain to the gastrocnemius-soleus complex and Achilles tendon. Hill workouts should be done at a maximum once a week to allow the body time to heal. Similar to any chronic injury to the feet, shoes must be evaluated. Athletes need to learn and understand their foot type and the proper shoes for their foot type. Also, shoes should be replaced every 500 miles are a maximum 2 years. Running on old worn shoes will alter biomechanics and cause stress and strain to the body. Finally, the lack of flexibility is often the main culprit in Achilles tendonitis. The importance of stretching and stretching often should be emphasized.

Prophylactic Support

Initially, heel cups will reduce the tension and stress placed on the Achilles tendon. As flexibility is regained, the heel cup should be gradually reduced to reduce the chances of an adaptive shortening of the tendon. Athletes may find comfort in a special tape job that will reduce the stress placed on the Achilles tendon as well. The patient's foot type and gait mechanics should be evaluated for possible use of custom orthotics. Achilles tendonitis can often be attributed to over pronation during gait. A custom orthotic will be able to adjust the athlete's gait to reduce this abnormality.

Turf Toe

Tuft toe is a hyperextension injury of the great toe, causing a sprain to the metatarsophalangeal joint and damage to the joint capsule. Turf toe can be either an acute or a chronic condition. An acute turf toe often occurs when the athlete's shoe sticks into the ground while he/she is trying to stop quickly. The shoe sticks as the individual's body weight shifts forward, causing the big toe to jam into the shoe and ground. The chronic condition occurs from frequent running or jumping in shoes that allow excessive great toe motion. This mechanism of injury may occur on natural or synthetic surfaces.

Athletes with turf toe will present with pain at the 1st metatarsophalangeal joint. Swelling and stiffness may be present, however pain, especially with great toe extension is the primary symptom. Rehabilitation of turf toe typically requires several weeks. If left untreated, turf toe can lead to permanent decrease in range of motion and osteoarthritis arthritis.

Rehabilitation Concerns

Patients suffering from turf toe respond best with rest and an adjustment made to their shoes. Pain management should be of primary concern to the clinician. Once pain and swelling have been reduced, the athlete should start performing toe extension and flexion exercises such as toe crunches and short foot exercises. Joint mobilizations should be added to the treatment protocol to aid in pain and increase range of motion. Once pain and swelling is reduced, the athlete may begin to progress into athletic activities. Protecting the great toe with a stiff forefoot insert or a great toe taping may increase athlete comfort.

Criteria for Full Competition

Athletes are able to return to full competition when any pain and swelling has resolved. Often athletes with turf toe are capable to continue practicing and participating while suffering from this injury with the toe being taped and possible inserts into shoes.

Pearls of Wisdom

- Have patients wear stiff insoled shoes to prevent excessive motion.

- Great toe joint mobilizations can be incorporated to reduce pain and increase motion.

Patient Education

Patients should be aware that if left untreated, turf toe may cause permanent decreased range of motion in the great toe and bone spurs may develop. Although athletes can often play with turf toe, rest and pain management is the most beneficial for athletes. Without prevention of excessive extension of the great toe, symptoms of turf toe may disappear with rest just to return once the athlete returns to activity.

Prophylactic Support

Athletes with turf toe may benefit from adding a steel or other stiff material insert into the forefoot of the shoes to reduce extension. Taping of the great toe to prevent dorsiflexion may also be done.

Sports Concussion

Sport-related concussions are a complex pathophysiological process affecting the brain, induced by acute traumatic biomechanical forces. Concussions typically result in short-lived neurological impairments that resolve spontaneously and most often do not involve loss of consciousness (LOC).

Concussions are typically caused by a direct blow to the head, face, neck or elsewhere on the body with an "impulsive" force transmitted to the head from an opposing player, stationary object, or the ground.

There are an estimated 1.6-3.8 million sport-related concussions in the U.S. each year. Recent data suggest a trend of increased annual concussion rates over the past decade, which is speculated to be a result of the emphasis on concussion education and awareness leading to increased identification and reporting. Actual incidence may be higher, with studies showing up to 50% of concussions going unreported. Sports with the highest risk appear to be football and girl's soccer. Other high-risk sports include ice hockey and lacrosse. History of a previous concussion is a clear risk factor. In sports with similar rules for each gender, the incidence is higher in females, but there is insufficient evidence to clearly state that females are at higher risk. Although it is felt that younger athletes may need more conservative management, there is insufficient data to conclude that age is a risk factor for concussion.

Patho-Anatomy/Physiology

A concussion occurs from either a direct blow to the brain, or from an indirect blow that results in shearing forces diffusely across the brain. After the impact, a metabolic cascade ensues, including the release of excitatory neurotransmitters from the brain, which leads to a hypermetabolic state which lasts from days to weeks. Free radicals are produced and cerebral perfusion is decreased.

Disease progression including natural history, disease phases or stages, disease trajectory.

The onset of symptoms following a concussion is typically immediate or within minutes after the initial impact. The most common reported symptoms are headache and dizziness. Acutely, the athlete may also describe a feeling of fogginess, complain of tinnitus, confusion, flashing lights, nausea, or amnesia. Other commonly reported symptoms are sensitivity to bright lights, altered sleep patterns, poor concentration, and irritability. In addition, an athlete may notice increasing fatigue and delayed reaction time with physical and mental tasks. Long-term effects might include neurobehavioral or cognitive impairments.

Following a sports concussion, there is typically a step-wise gradual reduction in symptoms. The majority of concussions resolve within 7 to 10 days, but some cases may evolve to postconcussion syndrome (PCS) through a process that is poorly understood. PCS is defined as symptoms and signs of concussion that persist for weeks to months after the incident. Management is similar to acute concussion, and the foundation is time.

Specific Secondary or Associated Conditions and Complications

Complications of a concussion in the absence of other significant medical diagnoses or injuries are usually related to cognitive impairments. The athlete may experience insomnia, emotional lability, memory impairments, depression, anxiety, fatigue, headache, and dizziness.

Essentials of Assessment

It is essential to understand that direct head trauma is not necessary for a concussion to occur. After a suspected concussion, the athlete should be questioned on the incident that caused the impact and what current symptoms he/she is experiencing. A graded symptoms checklist provides a tool for the initial assessment and tracking of symptoms over subsequent evaluations. Symptoms include somatic (eg: headache), cognitive (eg: feeling like in a fog), sleep disturbance (insomnia) and/or emotional (eg: lability). The patient may not be able to recall the incident so other spectators may need to be questioned or game tapes reviewed.

Physical Examination

Initially, the on-field examination should focus on evaluating for emergent injuries. The cervical spine, skull and facial bones need to be palpated for any evidence of fracture. If the athlete is stable, a sideline assessment should be made. A thorough neurological evaluation needs to be performed that includes cranial nerves, sensation, strength, coordination, and balance. Maddocks questions are asked of the athlete, which test memory of details related to the current and past games. Cognitive assessment should be employed and should focus on immediate memory, concentration, and delayed recall. Standardized assessment tools are available, and they are designed to reduce the degree of subjectivity encountered by medical providers responsible for making a rapid and precise injury assessment and concussion diagnosis decision. When possible, sideline tests can be compared to a reliable preinjury baseline. Follow-up office examinations should include a graded symptom checklist, neurological exam, balance and coordination testing, as well as some form of cognitive assessment.

Functional Assessment

The athlete will often have cognitive deficits after sustaining a concussion. The length of the deficits can be highly variable. Concentration, attention, mood, and sleep can be affected, which can further impact school, work, and daily activities. The athlete's school performance should be closely followed after a concussion. A comprehensive neuropsychological evaluation can be used to identify subtle deficits.

Laboratory Studies

There are currently no recommendations for laboratory studies directly related to a concussion, unless there is concern for other clinically suspected pathology.

Imaging

Neuroimaging is typically normal after a player has sustained a sport-related concussion, and is therefore not recommended. Computed tomography (CT) scan and magnetic resonance imaging (MRI) should be reserved for those athletes suspected of intracranial pathology. Findings that would warrant neuroimaging include worsening mental status, declining level of consciousness, focal neurological deficits, seizures, intractable vomiting, anisocoria (not present prior to injury), rhinorrhea, or otorrhea. The use of functional MRI has shown correlation with symptom severity and recovery, but is not recommended for routine evaluation.

Supplemental Assessment Tools

Multiple tools can be used in the acute phase after a concussion; the one most recommended is the Sport Concussion Assessment Tool 3 (SCAT3). SCAT3 utilizes a multifaceted standardized method to evaluate an athlete with either a known or suspected concussion. It incorporates the Maddocks questions and the Standardized Assessment of Concussion (SAC), with assessments of symptom evaluation, loss of consciousness, Glasgow Coma Scale, cognition, balance, and coordination. Balance testing in SCAT3 utilizes the Balance Error Scoring System (BESS) in which single-leg, double-leg, and tandem stance is evaluated. SCAT3 can be used sequentially to track an athlete's recovery. While most concussions can be appropriately managed without a comprehensive instrumental neuropsychological evaluation, it can be used to identify subtle deficits and further guide management.

Early Predictions of Outcomes

Many studies have looked at predictors of outcomes following sports concussions and studies have been disparate. Recently, separate studies have suggested that presence of post-traumatic amnesia and symptoms of fogginess are associated with prolonged recovery. Youth athletes may have a more prolonged recovery and are more susceptible to a concussion accompanied by a catastrophic injury. A greater number, severity, and duration of symptoms after concussion are predictors of a prolonged recovery. History of pre-injury mood disorders, learning disorders, Attention Deficit Disorder/Attention Deficit Hyperactivity Disorder (ADD/ADHD), and migraine headache complicate diagnosis and management of concussion.

Social Role and Social Support System

Individuals may notice that attempting tasks in the home and at work/school often increase their concussive symptoms. For student athletes, teachers need to have the understanding that they may need additional time with homework or testing due to problems with attention and concentration. Cognitive rest is very important in the acute recovery from a concussion, and includes restrictions on cell phone use, texting, video games, physical activity and school work until symptoms abate.

Some athletes experience mood-related consequences including anxiety and depression. Contributing factors may include frustration over uncertain recovery time, isolation from teammates and sport, and lack of social support. Prior to pharmacologic or psychotherapy, treatment involves behavioral management interventions, such as regulated sleep schedule, proper nutrition and stress reduction. Helping the athlete to identify and talk about the etiology of the symptoms can be helpful.

Professional Issues

Returning a concussed athlete back to activities too soon after injury is the situation that needs to be avoided. Thus, the physiatrist must have a process in place to prevent this from happening. If athletes are returned to play prior to full recovery, both cognitively and physically, they are at risk for worsening symptoms, an increased risk of suffering additional concussions, and in the worst cases, second impact syndrome which results in severe brain swelling, significant morbidity and often death.

Rehabilitation Management and Treatments

Available or Current Treatment Guidelines

Return to play in sport is the key issue after a concussion and should occur only after medical clearance from a licensed health care provider trained in the evaluation and management of concussion. Return to play involves a 6-step program: 1. No activity, 2. Light aerobic exercise, 3. Sport specific exercise, 4. Non-contact training drills, 5. Full-contact practice, 6. Return to play. The athlete progresses to the next step when asymptomatic for 24 hours. If symptoms occur with activity, the progression should be halted and restarted at the preceding symptom-free step. Athletes should be off of medications that may mask or modify symptoms of concussion.

Different Disease Stages

On the sideline, the athlete should be removed from the field of play and not allowed to return if there a concussion suspected. The initial treatment after a concussion is physical and cognitive rest. The brain is in a hypermetabolic state after a concussion and physically demanding activities, in light of reduced cerebral perfusion, can increase symptoms and delay recovery. The athlete should avoid cognitive activities such as playing video games, watching television, and reading, as well as physically demanding activities which may exacerbate their symptoms. "Cognitive rest" with respect to academics may include a temporary leave of absence, shortened school days, reduced workloads, additional time for assignments and exams. Standardized testing during recovery is discouraged as scores may be lower than expected. Individuals should also avoid high-risk activities that may cause additional concussions and worsen symptoms even further. Over-the-counter melatonin may be prescribed for mild insomnia, or trazodone or amitriptyline for more severe cases. It is not uncommon for depression or anxiety to develop, for which prescribing an anti-depressant or anxiolytic can be considered if symptoms persist.

Coordination of Care

The approach to an athlete with a sport-related concussion should integrate many individuals. A physician familiar with sports concussions should be directing care and decisions, often involving collaboration with physical/occupational therapists and neuropsychologists. Additionally, athletic trainers, family, coaching staff, teachers, and friends also need to be a part of the treatment process.

Patient and Family Education

The athlete, family, friends, teachers and coaches need to be educated on the effects of sport-related concussion. There needs to be an understanding of the injury in order to protect the athlete and support him/her through the recovery process.

Emerging/Unique Interventions

Neuropsychological testing is the best measurement to evaluate cognitive impairment. This testing commonly utilizes computer-based programs that are simple and sensitive, but these are not substitutes for formal neuropsychologic testing. These computerized tests evaluate an athlete's visual memory, verbal memory, processing speed, and reaction time and can follow the resolution of cognitive deficits with serial testing. Although there is insufficient evidence to recommend the widespread routine use of baseline neuropsychological testing, this may be more important in high-risk athletes with a prior history of concussion, confounding conditions (learning disability, mood and attention disorders, migraine headaches), or those in high-risk sports.

The most important aspect of sport-related concussions is the removal of athletes from sports activities as they are recovering. There are many useful tools for monitoring symptoms and cognition to help aid in the decision on when the athlete is ready to return to full participation. Although computer-based neuropsychological testing is becoming a cornerstone of concussion management, written tests are more comprehensive (and time consuming).

Cutting Edge/Emerging and Unique Concepts and Practice

Concussion legislation has been emerging in this country since the state of Washington passed the first concussion bill in 2009, the Lystedt Law, which required athletes to be removed immediately from athletic activities if it is suspected they have sustained a concussion. Within 5 years, all 50 states have passed a similar law. In order to return to play, athletes must be evaluated and receive written clearance from a health care provider trained in concussion assessment.

There is increasing concern that head impact exposure and recurrent concussions contribute to long-term neurologic sequelae such as chronic neurological impairment. Some studies have suggested an association between previous concussions and chronic cognitive dysfunction. Chronic Traumatic Encephalopathy (CTE) represents a distinct tauopathy with an unknown incidence in the athletic populations. A cause and effect relationship has not as yet been demonstrated between CTE and concussions or exposure to contact sports.

A new emerging treatment for concussion is high dose omega-3 fatty acids, which may decrease neural inflammation caused by concussion. High dose fish oil administered to rats demonstrated a significant decrease in brain damage compared to rats that did not received supplementation.

Vestibular rehabilitation has been demonstrated to decrease dizziness and lead to improvement in balance quicker than athletes who did not undergo vestibular rehabilitation.

Genetic testing and blood tests for certain biomarkers to assist in treating concussions have some promise, but are not currently recommended for routine use. These include Apolipoprotein (Apo) E4, Tau polymerase, glial fibrillary acidic protein (GFAP), neuron specific enolase (NSE), and myelin basic protein (MBP).

Sports and Occupational Injuries to the Wrist and Hand

There is no universal definition of sports injury. In general, most studies examining sports injury consider an injury to be a loss or abnormality of structure or function sustained during an athletic activity that alters athletic performance and produces time loss from participation. It should be noted that that this definition is often sport- and athlete-specific. For a given defect in structure or function, there will not be equal loss of performance or participation amongst all sports or individual athletes.

Sports and occupational injuries may be broadly classified as occurring either from trauma or repetitive use. The underlying etiologic mechanism of injury is often dynamic, complex, and multifactorial.

In sports activities, acute hand and wrist injuries are often the result of falls, blunt force (i.e., helmet, ball, stick, or other player), rotational forces, and flexion/extension forces (i.e., grasping another player).

Wrist injuries account for 3.6% of work-related injuries with an incidence of 3.8/10,000 full time workers and an average of 14 days off work. Hand injuries account for 12.5%, with an incidence of 13.0/10,000 and an average of 5 days off work.

Although hand amputations account for 0.5% of all hand and wrist injuries, finger amputations account for 95% of all work-related amputations. The use of two-handed activation switches and guards to push materials into machinery has helped to reduce the incidence of amputation.

A majority of occupational illness is due to repeated trauma, and of these, musculoskeletal disorders of the hand and wrist are associated with longest absence from work and greatest lost productivity and wages. The onset and severity of work related musculoskeletal injuries of the hand and wrist is associated with forceful and repetitive hand use. These disorders are worsened by poor ergonomics or performing tasks in the presence of vibration or cold, and are also affected by psychosocial and non-workplace factors.

Hand and wrist injuries are common among athletes, with a rate of 3 to 9% among all sports. Many injuries remain unrecognized and/or under-reported by athletes, making it difficult to ascertain the true incidence. Overuse injuries constitute between 25-50% of hand and wrist injuries. Traumatic injuries vary by sport and position and are more prevalent in full contact and stick and ball/puck sports.

Athletes under age 16 show injury rates of 14.8% for upper extremity; 16% involving the hand and 9% the wrist. Eighty-five percent of sport hand fractures occur from football, basketball, and lacrosse, with football accounting for 50% of these.

Risk factors for sports injury include extrinsic factors such as playing surface, weather, equipment and protective gear, and other players as well as intrinsic factors such as training load, prior injury, and individual anatomy, biomechanics, and neuromuscular coordination. Primary prevention of hand and wrist injury in sport may be accomplished by modification of these risk factors. For example, there is potential for reduction in injury incidence through advances in equipment technology, rule changes, and improved technique and training protocols.

Patho-Anatomy/Physiology

Subtle injuries can be missed without detailed knowledge of anatomy.

Triangular Fibrocartilage Complex (TFCC) injury involves tears of the fibrocartilage articular disc and tissue that connects the disc to the triquetrum and other carpals. The TFCC acts as the primary stabilizer to the distal radioulnar joint and cushions articulations between the ulnar head and the lunate and triquetrum.

The ulnar collateral ligament (UCL) of the thumb is an important stabilizer. The term "Gamekeeper's Thumb" refers to a chronic injury of the UCL usually acquired through repeated low-grade hyperabduction. The term "Skier's Thumb" refers to an acute tear or sprain of the UCL that often occurs with abrupt, forceful thumb stress in extension and/or abduction (i.e., skiing injuries, football, judo). A Stener lesion occurs when the UCL ruptures from the base of the proximal phalanx and retracts proximally. The proximal end of the UCL becomes lodged between the adductor pollicis aponeurosis, preventing healing. Surgery is required to prevent permanent instability.

Scapholunate dissociations are seen following a fall onto an outstretched, dorsally extended and ulnar deviated wrist, causing scapholunate ligament tear and dorsal shift. With more forceful trauma, there can be disassociation between the capitate and/or triquetrum.

The proximal interphalangeal (PIP) joint is a hinge joint that is stabilized by both the bony anatomy and by collateral, dorsal, and volar ligaments. Injuries of the PIP joint range from mild sprains to complex fractures. PIP joint dislocations occur when there is traumatic disruption of the thick volar ligament and at least one of the collateral ligaments. The volar ligament is the primary palmar PIP joint stabilizer preventing hyperextension, and dorsal dislocations are the most common.

Finger tendon injuries can involve disruption to the pulley system, resulting in instability/imbalance. Central slip of the extensor tendon over the PIP joint leads to boutonniere deformity, with lumbricals acting as flexors at the PIP and extending the DIP without opposing forces. Collateral ligament injury, usually at the PIP, can leads to PIP instability when the PIP is in 30 degrees of flexion and the metacarpal phalangeal joint (MCP) is flexed. Extensor tendon injury at the distal interphalangeal joint (DIP) from sudden passive flexion when the finger is extended causes mallet finger. Extensor tendon rupture and avulsion from the distal phalanx results in no active extension of the DIP in mallet finger. Finger flexor injury to the flexor digitorum profundus (jersey finger) leads to inability to flex the DIP joint. Volar plate injury commonly involves the PIP and collateral ligament following hyperextension of a finger joint.

Scaphoid fractures and dislocations are important to recognize due to the vascular supply of the scaphoid. Blood supply is received from the dorsal vessels of the radial artery and from the palmar and superficial palmar branches of the radial artery. Seventy to 80 percent of the bone (including the entire proximal pole) is supplied from branched dorsal vessels. The tubercle and distal end of the scaphoid is supplied by palmar vessels. Fracture to the middle and proximal portions are at risk for nonunion and osteonecrosis.

Distal radius fractures are typically caused by a fall on outstretched hand. There are several subtypes of distal radius fracture that can be broadly classified as intra-articular, partially articular, or completely articular. The Colles fracture is one of the most common subtypes, and describes a dorsally angulated and displaced extra-articular distal radius fracture.

Hook of hamate and pisiform fractures occur with either repetitive stress or sudden, forceful impact. They are usually seen in athletes who handle a racquet, bat, club, or stick, almost exclusively in the leading hand.

Metacarpal fractures occur typically due to trauma with a fall on outstretched hand or direct blow from contact.

Median nerve entrapment syndromes can occur from anatomical reduction of carpal tunnel space. Dorsal or volar lunate dislocation from high energy injury, and distal radial fractures can affect the median nerve.

Disease progression including natural history, disease phases or stages, disease trajectory.

Treatment is guided by severity. Milder injuries may be treated with protected activity, supportive splinting or casting, inflammation control, and gradual return to activity. Occasionally residual soft tissue stiffness occurs. Stretching and motion exercises to minimize mobility loss is important.

Sub-acute pain may present with movement loss around the injured structure, caused by soft tissue stiffness from scarring, ongoing inflammation, or weakened surrounding muscles. Therapy is recommended to prevent stiffness, strengthen weakened muscles and improve range of motion and alleviate patient fears of moving the injured structure. Exercises, ultrasound, electrical stimulation, massage or other modalities help recovery. Medication can be used at to control pain or inflammation. Gradually range of motion may return to normal.

Unrecognized or untreated soft tissue injuries may result in instability leading to progressive cartilage degeneration and arthritis. Arthritic changes may result in pain, stiffness, and swelling; symptoms may be intermittent and vary in severity. Chronic mild or intermittent symptoms may be treated with splinting, activity modifications, and analgesics or anti-inflammatory medications. Significant symptom flare may be treated with steroid injection.

Specific Secondary or Associated Conditions and Complications

Complications of sports injuries of the hand and wrist can result in significant including longer time away from sport and potentially long-term disability. Accurate and timely diagnosis is important in establishing the correct treatment. Iatrogenic injury must be avoided during both surgical and non-surgical treatments.

Distal radius fractures may provoke extensor pollicis longus tenosynovitis or rupture. Undiagnosed scaphoid fractures may lead to scaphoid non-union advanced collapse, resulting in need for arthroplasty.

Delayed diagnosis of hook of hamate fracture may lead to complications, including flexor tendon rupture. Ulnar neuropathy may be associated with fracture of the hamate or pisiform. Due to the anatomy of the ulnar nerve around Guyon's canal, this may present as a pure sensory, pure motor, or mixed sensory and motor deficit.

Intra-articular fractures of the metacarpals at the CMC joint can cause long-term pain or dysfunction, even with operative management. Instability of the thumb following intra-articular fracture may require CMC arthrodesis for the athlete to regain stability. Stener lesion of the thumb UCL requires surgical assessment.

Untreated scapholunate interosseous injuries may develop a pattern of degenerative arthritis known as scapholunate advanced collapse. PIP ligament injuries and PIP dislocation often result in suboptimal outcomes due to a lack of recognition of the seriousness of injury. Overtreatment with prolonged immobilization can also cause long-term dysfunction.

Improper management of tendon injuries may result in permanent deformity and dysfunction.

Essentials of Assessment

Mechanism of injury is the most important in diagnosis. History of high velocity or rotational stress injury versus pain after repetitive strain quickly narrows the diagnosis. For example, a fall on an outstretched hand (FOOSH) can cause scaphoid, distal radius fractures or damage the TFCC. Also, rotational stress to the wrist may cause a tear in the TFCC.

Pain location (dorsal, volar, ulnar, or radial) and aggravating factors should be assessed. Pain after repeated movements with stiffness after rest suggests inflammatory conditions. Night pain is often found in carpal tunnel syndrome. Pain exacerbated immediately following activities or increasing insidiously with activity should be noted. Acute onset versus gradual onset of pain can be helpful in further delineating the differential diagnosis. For example gradual-onset pain should make you consider systemic conditions causing pain in hand or wrist.

Presence, location (diffuse or localized) and severity of swelling and a history of acute swelling following an injury, versus gradual swelling, help to identify repetitive conditions from residuals of acute trauma. A history of previous injuries or surgeries may affect the symptoms of the injury.

Complaints of changes in sensation and color may aid in determining neurovascular involvement. Crepitus, degree of pain, bruising, and/or loss of function must be documented. Joint clicking may be associated with carpal instability, triangular fibrocartilage tears, or extensor carpi ulnaris subluxation.

Other important, yet often forgotten, aspects of the history are hand dominance, occupation and presence of recurrent wrist swelling.

Physical Examination

First observe for any swelling, ecchymosis, gross deformity or atrophy (such as thenar or hypothenar wasting). Also observe for how the patient is holding the wrist or hand as well as any scars or skin changes. Often testing both active and passive range of motion of the wrist and fingers can show functional deficits that will help you focus your exam. Identify movements and positions that cause pain or discomfort. Pain from stretching shortened contractile tissues occurs at the end range of passive motion. Active movements employ contractile tissues, while also moving inert tissues in the process. Palpation of the wrist and fingers is imperative especially when there is concern for scaphoid fracture, Dupuytren's contracture, trigger finger or 1 carpometacarpal joint arthritis. Strength testing will help elucidate any focal weakness that could be caused by carpal tunnel syndrome or ulnar neuropathy.

Special Tests

For Ligament, Capsule and Joint Instability

Thumb Ulnar Collateral Ligament Stress Test or Finger Collateral Ligament Stress Test assesses digit ligamentous stability. Murphy's sign is indicative of a lunate dislocation demonstrated by the patient making a fist and observing the distal end of the 3rd metacarpal in relation to the 2nd and 4th. Supination Lift test can help the examiner determine if there is TFCC pathology present. Axial Load test identifies possible metacarpophalangeal joint arthrosis and possible fracture of the metacarpals or adjacent bones. Watson test and/or a Shuck test identify scapholunate dissociation.

For Tendons and Muscles

Finkelstein test for Dequervain's tenosynovitis or Axial Grind Test for carpal metacarpal (CMC) arthritis evaluate for thumb pain. Elson test and Boye's test identify extensor digitorum central slip injuries. Sweater finger sign or Flexor Digitorum Profundus test identify possible rupture of the tendon or avulsion of the tendon from the phalanx attachment.

For Neurologic Dysfunction

Finger opposition to the thumb and opening and closing the hand requires normal joint function, normal functioning flexor and extensor tendons, and intact median and ulnar nerves. Carpal Compression, Tinel test at the wrist or Phalen test identify possible carpal tunnel syndrome. Froment sign or Tinel test at the elbow and Ulnar Compression Test will aid in the evaluation of possible ulnar neuropathy. ling's maneuver for assessing nerve root pain. Referred pain originating from the cervical spine or other proximal structures must be considered.

Other Special Tests

Testing grip provides an objective measurement of the integrity and strength of intrinsic hand and forearm muscles. A grip dynamometer is accurate and reproducible.

Functional Assessment

Emotional reactions, such as a lack of confidence, apprehension, and fear can play a role in an athletes ability to return to play. These reactions may become problematic, interfering with performance, and increasing the probability of re-injury. The physician should not only evaluate physical factors in determining return to play readiness, but also consider psychological well-being.

Laboratory Studies

In patients recalcitrant to treatment, workup for other conditions needs to be considered. Elevated erythrocyte sedimentation rate (ESR) and C-reactive protein (CRP) are nonspecific tests that are associated with inflammatory causes of pain. These labs are non-specific but may indicate inflammatory rheumatic disease, especially if only a modest degree of inflammation is present. Rheumatoid factors are often seen elevated in patients with Rheumatoid Arthritis, but can also be seen in other disease processes such as Sjögren's syndrome, and Systemic Lupus Erythematosus.

Imaging

For wrist injury, X-ray in neutral as well as PA with both radial and ulnar deviation, are recommended.

Scapholunate instability cannot be ruled out on initial plain radiographs because it may take months for scaphoid and lunate to separate significantly radiographically.

Ultrasound is a quick way to assess soft tissue abnormality such as tendon issues, synovial thickening, ganglions, and synovial cyst.

MRI may be equally sensitive to and more specific than a bone scan for fracture, and provide information about soft tissue structures.

Supplemental Assessment Tools

The Patient-Rated Wrist and Hand Evaluation (PRWHE) is a 15-item self-reported questionnaire about pain and disability that can be used to evaluate outcome after hand injuries.

A dynamometer evaluates grip strength and helps evaluate for possible disuse atrophy, arthritis, carpal tunnel syndrome, epicondylitis, and decreased motor function due to radiculopathy.

A Purdue pegboard dexterity test can be used to measure dexterity for activities that involve gross movements of the arms, wrists, hands, and fingers.

Social Role and Social Support System

Poor coping can preclude recovery. Patients can develop new psychosocial needs that are not adequately addressed. Social support patterns can change with increased reliance on coaches, trainers and medical team members. Loss of confidence and emotional stressors may require different strategies (i.e., goal setting and mental imagery) to provide positive psychological support.

Rehabilitation Management and Treatments

Many hand and finger injuries require specific rehabilitation and appropriate protection on resumption of sport. Joints in this area do not respond well to immobilization and therefore full immobilization should be minimized.

Decision when to return to play is individualized and depends a variety of factures including health status of individual, participation risk, and external influences. Risks of return to play will vary with each sport, and external influences include family, team, legal and financial considerations.

Stable phalangeal and metacarpal fractures treated non-operatively may have protected return to play before 4 weeks. Whereas, unprotected return is typically between 4 to 8 weeks depending on risks of the sport. Imaging should be obtained to ensure adequate healing has occurred before unprotected return to play is allowed. Similar guidelines are followed for surgically corrected fractures but risk vs benefit must be considered by the surgeon. Acceptable protective devices vary and are determined by each sport's governing body.

Exceptions for return to play following fracture include scaphoid fractures. Return to play can occur 4 weeks after injury without increased risk of nonunion. Typically, between 8 to 12 weeks of immobilization is required before attempting unprotected return to play with nonoperative scaphoid fractures. There is a wide variation of 2 to 12 weeks for return to play after surgical fixation of scaphoid fractures. This depends on risks related to each individual sport.

Ligamentous injuries have a similar return to play timeline as fractures. UCL, scapholunate ligament, and mallet injuries may return to sport immediately with protection for 4 to 6 weeks. Jersey fingers are treated surgically and require significant healing time of up to 4 months before return to contact sports.

Different Disease Stages

Functional rehabilitation requires mobility, stability, sensitivity, and freedom from pain. Coordinated management can effectively address these needs during different phases of recovery. During the inflammatory phase, edema and pain reduction edema are essential. Control of edema can be achieved through splinting, compression, ice, elevation, and electrotherapeutic modalities. In the regenerative phase, there is a pro-liferation of scar tissue. Therapists can use supportive splints and active exercises to maintain range of motion. In the remodeling phase, dynamic and serial splints, as well as active assist exercises in addition to heat, stretching, and electrotherapeutic modalities are employed.

Coordination of Care

Patients with occupational and sports injuries often require input from various disciplines (medical, therapy, training and psychological intervention) to achieve optimal outcomes. Communication and sharing of information among all participants concerned with a patient's care achieve safer and more effective care.

Patient and Family Education

The patient and the social support network (family, friends, significant others) should play a part in the multi-disciplinary approach to helping achieve the goals and needs of the patient.

Emerging/Unique Interventions

The Disabilities of the Arm, Shoulder and Hand (DASH) questionnaire is a 30-item questionnaire that looks at the ability of a patient to perform certain upper extremity activities, allowing patients to rate difficulty and interference with daily life on a 5-point Likert scale.

The QuickDASH is an abbreviated version of the original DASH outcome measure and contains only 11 items.

Translation into practice: practice "pearls"/performance improvement in practice (pips)/changes in clinical practice behaviors and skills.

Work-related prognosis often is not based on pathology but on other factors.

Cutting Edge/Emerging and Unique Concepts and Practice

The use of Orthobiologics is an emerging paradigm for the treatment of wrist and hand conditions. Most orthobiologics being used for these conditions are Platelet Rich Plasma (PRP), Stem-cells and Autologous blood. These agents are being injected into the hand and wrist for conditions including tendinopathies, arthritis, chondropathies as well as instability injuries.

Recently the injection of steroids and anesthetic agents into and around cartilaginous structures has been called into question. There is some evidence to suggest that these agents are causing cartilage and tendon damage especially with repeated injections. Their use is being called into question especially with the rise of orthobiologics.

Shin-Splint Syndrome

Medial Tibial Stress Syndrome (MTSS) or Shin-Splint Syndrome is a clinical pain condition defined as exercise-induced pain along the posteromedial tibial border (distal third) caused by repetitive loading stress during running and jumping and provoked on palpation over a length of ≥5consecutive centimeters.

Another proposed terminology is that, "A more descriptive term that explains the inflammatory traction event in the tibial aspect of the common leg in the runners is the medial periostitis of the tibial traction or simply the tibial periostitis medial".

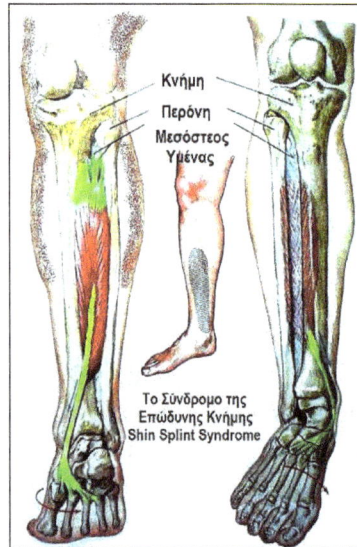

Clinically Relevant Anatomy

The pathophysiology of shin splints is more easily understood after examining the relevant cross-sectional anatomy. There are 4 muscle compartments in the leg:

- Anterior: This compartiment contains the tibialis anterior muscle, the extensor hallucis longus, the extensor digitorum longus and the peroneus tertius.

    ◦ The tibialis anterior dorsiflexes the ankle and inverts the foot.

    ◦ The extensor hallucis longus extends the great toe.

    ◦ The extensor digitorum longus extends the other toes and assists in eversion as does the peroneus tertius.

- Deep posterior: This contains the flexor digitorum longus, the tibialis posterior and the flexor hallucis longus.

    ◦ The tibialis posterior plantar flexes and inverts the foot.

- ○ The others are predominantly toe flexors.

- Superficial posterior: this is the gastrocnemius and soleus group; predominatly plantar flexors of the ankle.

- Lateral: this compartment contains the peroneus brevis and longus, mainly foot evertors.

A dysfunction of tibialis anterior and posterior are commonly implicated, also the area of attachment of these muscles can be the location of pain. Muscle imbalance and inflexibility, especially tightness of the triceps surae (gastrocnemius, soleus, and plantaris muscles), is commonly associated with MTSS. Athletes with muscle weakness of the triceps surae are more prone to muscle fatigue, leading to altered running mechanics, and strain on the tibia. Clinicians should also examine for inflexibility and imbalance of the hamstring and quadriceps muscles.

Epidemiology/Etiology

Shin splint is a common overuse sports injury with incidence rates from 4% to 19% in athletic populations and 4% to 35% of military population.

In runners (sprinters, middle and long distance runners and footballers) has been identified as the most common-related musculoskeletal injury with an incidence rate ranging from 13.6% to 20.0% and a prevalence of 9.5%. Also in dancers it is present in 20% of the population and up to 35% of the new recruits of runners and dancers will develop it.

Shin-splints is most common with running and jumping athletes who made training errors, especially when they overload or when they run too fast for their potential. This injury can also be related to changes in the training program, such as an increase in distance, intensity and duration. Running on a hard or uneven surface and bad running shoes (like a poor shock absorbing capacity) could be one of the factors related to the casualty. Biomechanical abnormalities as foot arch abnormalities, hyperpronation of the foot, unequal leg length, are the most frequently mentioned intrinsic factors.

Women have an increased risk to incur stress fractures, especially with this syndrome. This is due to nutrional, hormonal and biomechanical abnormalities. Individuals who are overweight are more susceptible to getting this syndrome. Therefore it is important that people who are overweight, combine their exercise with a diet or try to lose weight before starting therapy or a training program. These people, along with poor conditioned individuals, should always slowly increase their training level. Cold weather contributes to this symptom, therefore it's important (even more than usual) to warm up properly.

The pathophysiology is unclear but there are two hypothesis for discussion: periostitis induced by fascial traction or a local bone stress reaction. Internally a chronic inflammation of the muscular attachment along the posterior medial tibia and bony changes are considered to be the most likely cause of the medial tibial stress syndrome.

Characteristics/Clinical Presentation

The main symptom is dull pain at the distal two third of the posteromedial tibial border. The pain is non-focal but extends over "at least 5 cm" and is often bilateral. It also worsens at each moment of contact. A mild edema in this painful area may also be present and tenderness on palpation is typically present following the inducing activity for up to several days.

At first the patient only feels pain at the beginning of the workout, often disappearing while exercising, only to return during the cool-down period. When shin splints get worse the pain can remain during exercise and also could be present for hours of days after cessation of the inducing activity.

The most common complication of shin-splints is a stress fracture, which shows itself by tenderness of the anterior tibia. Neurovascular signs and symptoms are not commonly attributable to MTSS and when present, other pathologies such as chronic exertional compartment syndrome (CECS) or vascular deficiencies should be considered as the source of leg pain.

Differential Diagnosis

An algorithmic approach has been established for further differentiating exercise-induced leg pain entities:

- Pain at rest with palpable tenderness indicates bone stress injuries (MTSS and stress fractures).

- No pain at rest with palpable tenderness proposes nerve entrapment syndromes.

- No pain at rest with no palpable tenderness makes functional popliteal artery entrapment syndrome and chronic exertional compartment syndrome likely.

MTSS may overlap with the diagnosis of deep posterior compartment syndrome but the critical point for differentiation is the longer lasting post-exercise pain when compared with deep posterior chronic exertional compartment syndrome.

Compared with stress fractures, the painful area extends over more than 5 cm on the distal two thirds of the medial tibial border.

Key points for assessment and management for mtss	
History	Increasing pain during exercise related to the medial tibial border in the middle and lower third. Pain persists for hours or days after cessation of activity .
Physical examination	Intensive tenderness of the involved medial tibial border. More than 5 cm.
Imaging	MRI: Periosteal reaction and edema.
Treatment	Mainly conservative (running retraining, ESWT).

It is important to differentiate MTSS from:

• Stress Fracture,

• Chronic Exertional Compartmental Syndrome,

• Sciatica,

• Deep Vein Thrombosis (DVT),

• Popliteal Artery Entrapment,

• Muscle Strain,

• Tumour,

• Arterial endofibrosis,

• Infection,

• Nerve entrapment (common/superficial peroneus and saphenous).

The following are two conditions that are sometimes mistakenly diagnosed as shin splints.

Pain on the anterior (outside) part of the lower leg may be compartment syndrome: Swelling of muscles within a closed compartment which creates pressure. The symptoms of compartment syndrome include leg pain, unusual nerve sensations, and eventually muscle weakness.

Pain in the lower leg could also be a stress fracture (an incomplete crack in the bone), which is a far more serious injury than shin splints. The pain of a stress fracture is focal with tenderness in less than 5 cm. that can be find with a fingerprint as a definite spot of sharp pain. Additionally, stress fractures often feel better in the morning because the bone has rested all night; shin splints often feel worse in the morning because the soft tissue tightens overnight. Shin splints are also at their most painful when patient forcibly try to lift the foot up at the ankle and flex the foot.

Diagnostic Procedures

Making the diagnosis based on history and physical examination is the most logical approach.

- A standardised history include questions on the onset and location of the pain:

  - If there is exercise-induced pain along the distal 2/3 of the medial tibial border: MTSS diagnosis is suspected.

  - The athlete is asked of what aggravated and relieved their pain: If pain is provoked during or after physical activity and reduced with relative rest, MTSS diagnosis is suspected.

  - The athlete is asked about cramping, burning and pressure-like calf pain and/ or pins and needles in the foot (their presence could be signs of chronic exertional compartment syndrome, which could be a concurrent injury or the sole explanation for their pain): If no present, MTSS diagnosis is suspected.

- Physical examination If MTSS is suspected after the history: the posteromedial tibial border is palpated and the athletes are asked for the presence of recognisable pain (ie, from painful activities).

  - If no pain on palpation is present, or the pain is palpated over less than 5 cm: other lower leg injuries (eg, a stress fracture) has to be considered to be present and the athlete is labelled as not having MTSS.

  - If other symptoms not typical of MTSS are present (severe and visible swelling or erythema along the medial border): other leg injury should be considered.

  - If recognisable pain is present on palpation over 5 cm or more and no atypical symptoms are present, the diagnosis MTSS is confirmed.

Detmer in 1986 developed a classification system to subdivide MTSS into three types:

- Type I - Tibial microfracture, bone stress reaction or cortical fracture

- Type II - Periostalgia from chronic avulsion of the periosteum at the periosteal-fascial junction

- Type lll – Chronic compartment syndrome.

Imaging studies are not necessary to diagnose shin-splints, but when a conservative treatment fails, it could be useful to undertake an echo. If the injury has evolved into a stress fracture, an x-ray scan can show black lines. A triple-phase bone scan can show the difference between a stress fracture and a medial tibial stress syndrome. The MRI can also exclude tumors/edemas.

It is important that clinicians be aware that about 1/3 (32%) of the athletes with MTSS have co-existing lower leg injuries·

Outcome Measures

The MTSS score should be used as a primary outcome measure in MTSS because is valid, reliable and responsive. It measures:

- Pain at rest.

- Pain while performing activities of daily living.

- Limitations in sporting activities.

- Pain while performing sporting activities.

The MTSS score specifically measures pain along the shin and limitations due to shin pain.

Examination

Examination demonstrates an intensive tenderness on palpation along the medial tibial border, the anterior tibia, however, is usually nontender. Neurovascular symptoms are usually absent. Different from stress fracture, the pain is not focused to a specific point but covers a variable distance of several centimeters in the distal medial and proximal distal third of the tibia. In the painful area, there is no real muscle origin, but the deep crural fascia is attached to the medial tibial border. From clinical experience, a painful transverse band can frequently be palpated which most probably corresponds to the soleal aponeurosis.Therefore, MTSS is currently hypothesized to originate from tibial bone overload and not from adjacent soft tissue stress.

Physicians should carefully evaluate for possible knee abnormalities (especially genu varus or valgus), tibial torsion, femoral anteversion, foot arch abnormalities, or a leg-length discrepancy. Ankle movements and subtalar motion should also be evaluated. Clinicians should also examine for inflexibility and imbalance of the hamstring and quadriceps muscles and weakness of "core muscles". Core and pelvic muscle stability may be assessed by evaluating patient's ability to maintain a controlled, level pelvis during a pelvic bridge from the supine position, or a standing single-leg knee bend. Examining patient's shoes may reveal generally worn-out shoes or patterns consistent with a leg-length discrepancy or other biomechanical abnormalities. Abnormal gait patterns should be evaluated with the patient walking and running on a treadmill.

Physical Therapy Management

Patient education and a graded loading exposure program seem the most logical treatments. Conservative therapy should initially aim to correct functional, gait, and biomechanical overload factors. Recently 'running retraining' has been advocated as a promising treatment strategy and graded running programme has been suggested as a gradual tissue-loading intervention.

Prevention of MTSS was investigated in few studies and shock-absorbing insoles, pronation control insoles, and graduated running programs were advocated.

Overstress avoidance is the main preventive measure of MTSS or shin-splints. The main goals of shin-splints treatment are pain relieve and return to painfree activities.

For the treatment of shin-splints it's important to screen the risk factors, this makes it easier to make a diagnosis and to prevent this disease. In the next table you can find them.

Intrinsic Factors:

- Age,
- Sex,
- Height,
- Weight,
- Body fat,
- Femoral neck anteversion,
- Genu valgus,
- Pes clavus,
- Hyperpronation,
- Joint laxity,
- Aerobic endurance/conditioning,
- Fatigue,
- Strength of and balance between,
- flexors and extensors,
- Flexibility of muscles/joints,

- Sporting skill/coordination,

- Physiological factors.

Extrinsic Factors

- Sports-related factors,

- Type of sport,

- Exposure (e.g., running on one side of the road),

- Nature of event (e.g., running on hills),

- Equipment,

- Shoe/surface interface,

- Venue/supervision,

- Playing surface,

- Safety measures,

- Weather conditions,

- Temperature.

Control of risk factors could be a relevant strategy to initially avoid and treat MTSS: MIO2.

- Female gender,

- Previous history of MTSS,

- Fewer years of running experience,

- Orthotic use,

- Increased body mass index,

- Pronated foot posture (increased navicular drop),

- Increased ankle plantarflexion,

- Increased hip external rotation.

The role of hip internal rotation motion is unclear. Differences between hip muscle performance in MTSS and control subjects might be the effect rather than the cause MIO2.

Acute Phase

2-6 weeks of rest combined with medication is recommended to improve the symptoms and for a quick and safe return after a period of rest. NSAIDs and Acetaminophen are often used for analgesia. Also cryotherapy with Ice-packs and eventually analgesic gels can be used after exercise for a period of 20 minutes.

There are a number of physical therapy modalities to use in the acute phase but there is no proof that these therapies such as ultrasound, soft tissue mobilization, electrical stimulation would be effective. A corticoid injection is contraindicated because this can give a worse sense of health. Because the healthy tissue is also treated. A corticoid injection is given to reduce the pain, but only in connection with rest. Prolonged rest is not ideal for an athlete.

Subacute Phase

The treatment should aim to modify training conditions and to address eventual biomechanical abnormalities. Change of training conditions could be decreased running distance, intensity and frequency and intensity by 50%. It is advised to avoid hills and uneven surfaces.

During the rehabilitation period the patient can do low impact and cross-training exercises (like running on a hydro-gym machine).). After a few weeks athletes may slowly increase training intensity and duration and add sport-specific activities, and hill running to their rehabilitation program as long as they remain pain-free. A stretching and strengthening (eccentric) calf exercise program can be introduced to prevent muscle fatigue. (Level of Evidence: 3a) (Level of Evidence: 3a) (Level of Evidence: 5). Patients may also benefit from strengthening core hip muscles. Developing core stability with strong abdominal, gluteal, and hip muscles can improve running mechanics and prevent lower-extremity overuse injuries.

Proprioceptive balance training is crucial in neuromuscular education. This can be done with a one-legged stand or balance board. Improved proprioception will increase the efficiency of joint and postural-stabilizing muscles and help the body react to running surface incongruities, also key in preventing re-injury.

Choossing good shoes with good shock absorption can help to prevent a new or re-injury. Therefore it is important to change the athlete's shoes every 250-500 miles, a distance at which most shoes lose up to 40% of their shock-absorbing capabilities.

In case of biomechanical problems of the foot may individuals benefit from orthotics. An over-the-counter orthosis (flexible or semi-rigid) can help with excessive foot pronation and pes planus. A cast or a pneumatic brace can be necessary in severe cases.

Manual therapy can be used to control several biomechanical abnormalities of the spine, sacro-illiacal joint and various muscle imbalances. They are often used to prevent relapsing to the old injury.

There is also acupuncture, ultrasound therapy injections and extracorporeal shockwave therapy but their efficiency is not yet proved.

Rehabilitation of the Overhead Athlete's Elbow

Injuries to the elbow are common in the overhead athlete. Approximately 22% to 26% of all injuries to major league baseball pitchers involve the elbow joint. The repetitive overhead motion required of these athletes, in particular with throwing, is responsible for unique and sport-specific patterns of injuries to the elbow. Chronic stress overload or repetitive microtraumatic stress is observed during the overhead pitching motion as the elbow extends at over 2300 degrees per second, producing a medial shear force of 300 N and compressive force of 900 N. In addition, the valgus stress applied to the elbow during the acceleration phase of throwing is 64 Nm, exceeding the ultimate tensile strength of the ulnar collateral ligament (UCL). Thus, the medial aspect of the elbow undergoes tremendous tension (distraction) forces, while the lateral aspect is forcefully compressed during the throw. These forces may cause a variety of specific elbow injuries in this athletic population.

A number of forces act on the elbow during the act of throwing. These forces are maximal during the acceleration phase of throwing. Valgus stress in particular creates tensile forces across the medial aspect of the elbow, which may eventually cause tissue breakdown and the inability to throw. Compression forces are also applied to the lateral aspect of the elbow during the throwing motion. The posterior compartment is subject to tensile, compressive, and torsional forces during both the acceleration and deceleration phases, which may result in valgus extension overload within the posterior compartment, potentially leading to osteophyte formation, stress fractures of the olecranon, or physeal injury.

Rehabilitation following elbow injury or elbow surgery follows a sequential and progressive multiphased approach. The phases of the rehabilitation program should overlap to ensure proper progression. The ultimate goal of elbow rehabilitation is to return the athlete to his or her previous functional level as quickly and safely as possible.

Phase 1: Immediate Motion

The first phase of elbow rehabilitation is the immediate motion phase. The goals of this phase are to minimize the effects of immobilization, re-establish non-painful range of motion (ROM), decrease pain and inflammation, and retard muscular atrophy.

Early ROM activities are performed to nourish the articular cartilage and assist in the synthesis, alignment, and organization of collagen tissue. ROM activities are performed for all planes of elbow and wrist motions to prevent the formation of scar tissue and adhesions. Active-assisted and passive ROM exercises are performed at the humeroulnar joint to restore flexion/extension, as well as at both the humeroradial and radial-ulnar joints for supination/pronation. Reestablishing full elbow extension, typically defined as preinjury motion, is the primary goal of early ROM activities to minimize the occurrence of elbow flexion contractures.The preoperative elbow motion must be carefully assessed and recorded. Postoperatively, if the patient was not seen prior to injury or surgery, the athlete should be asked how much elbow extension had been present in the past 2 to 3 years. Attempting to compare elbow ROM to the contralateral side may not be adequate when restoring back to baseline.

The professional baseball pitcher often lacks approximately 3° to 5° of extension when tested in spring training physicals. The elbow is predisposed to flexion contractures due to the intimate congruency of the joint articulations, the tightness of the joint capsule, and the tendency of the anterior capsule to develop adhesions following injury. The brachialis muscle also attaches to the capsule and crosses the elbow joint before becoming a tendinous structure. Injury to the elbow may cause excessive scar tissue formation of the brachialis muscle as well as functional splinting of the elbow. Wright et al reported on 33 professional baseball players prior to the competitive season. The average loss of elbow extension was 7°, and the average loss of flexion was 5.5° compared to the opposite elbow joint. It is critical that postoperative ROM match preoperative motion, especially in the case of UCL reconstruction. This loss of extension can be a deleterious side effect for the overhead athlete.

Another goal of this phase is to decrease the patient's pain and inflammation. Cryotherapy, laser, and high-voltage stimulation may be needed to reduce pain and inflammation. Once the acute inflammatory response has subsided, moist heat, warm whirlpool, and ultrasound may be used at the onset of treatment to prepare the tissue for stretching and improve the extensibility of the capsule and musculotendinous structures. Grade I and II mobilization techniques may also be utilized in the early phases to neuromodulate pain by stimulating type I and type II articular receptors.

In addition to ROM exercises, joint mobilizations may be performed as tolerated to minimize the occurrence of joint contractures. Grade I and II mobilizations are initially used to help decrease pain and inflammation and later progressed to more aggressive grade III and IV mobilization techniques at end ROM, with the intended goal of improving ROM during later stages of rehabilitation when symptoms have subsided. Joint mobilization must include the radiocapitellar and radioulnar joints as well as maintain supination and pronation ROM. Posterior glides of the humeroulnar joint with oscillations are performed at end ROM to assist in regaining full elbow extension.

If the patient continues to have difficulty achieving full extension using ROM and mobilization techniques, a low-load, long-duration (LLLD) stretch may be performed to produce a deformation (creep) of the collagen tissue, resulting in tissue elongation. This technique appears to be extremely beneficial for regaining full elbow extension. The patient lies supine with a towel roll or a foam pad placed under the distal brachium to act as a cushion and fulcrum. Light-resistance exercise tubing is applied to the wrist of the patient and secured to the table or a dumbbell on the ground. The patient is instructed to relax as much as possible for 10 to 15 minutes per treatment. The resistance applied should enable the patient to stretch for the entire duration without pain or muscle spasm. This technique is intended to impart a low load during a long-duration stretch. Patients are instructed to perform the LLLD stretches several times per day, totaling at least 60 minutes of total end range time. We typically recommend a 15-minute stretch, 4 times per day. This program has been referred to as a TERT program (total end range time) and has been extremely beneficial for patients with a stiff elbow. However, in some patients who are not responding, splinting and bracing may be needed to create this LLLD stretch. This would require the patient to wear the brace at night for several hours while sleeping.

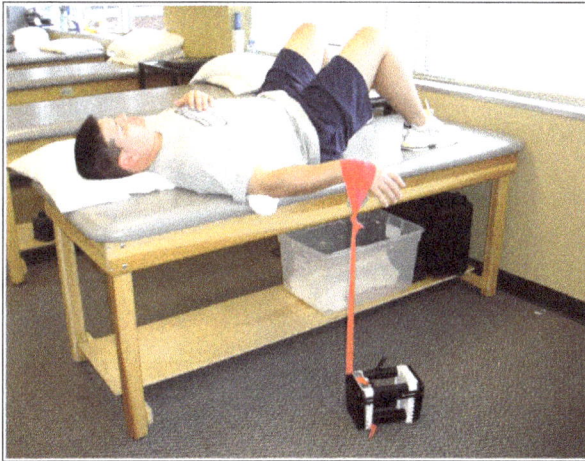

A low-load, long-duration stretch into elbow extension is performed using light resistance. The shoulder is internally rotated while the forearm is pronated to best isolate and maximize the stretch on the elbow joint.

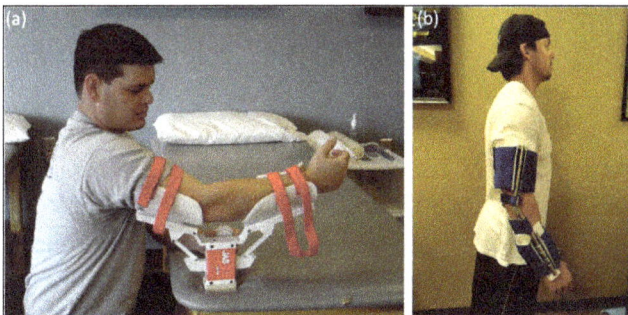

(a) Joint Active System (JAS, Effingham, Illinois) and (b) Dynasplint (Severna Park, Maryland) are 2 commercial devices commonly used by patients at home to work on elbow extension range of motion.

The aggressiveness of stretching and mobilization techniques is dictated by the healing constraints of involved tissues, as well as specific pathology/surgery and the amount of motion and end feel. For example, if the patient presents with a decrease in motion and hard end feel without pain, more aggressive stretching and mobilization technique may be used. Conversely, a patient exhibiting pain before resistance or an empty end feel will be progressed slowly with gentle stretching. In addition, it is beneficial to incorporate interventions to maintain proper glenohumeral joint ROM as indicated with each patient, including stretching and glenohumeral joint mobilizations.

The early phases of rehabilitation also focus on voluntary activation of muscle and retarding muscular atrophy. Subpainful and submaximal isometrics are performed initially for the elbow flexor and extensor, as well as the wrist flexor, extensor, pronator, and supinator muscle groups. Shoulder isometrics may also be performed during this phase with caution against internal and external rotation exercises, if painful, as the elbow joint becomes a fulcrum for shoulder isometrics. Scapular muscle strengthening is initiated immediately following the injury. Alternating rhythmic stabilization drills for shoulder flexion/extension/horizontal abduction/adduction, shoulder internal/external rotation, and elbow flexion/extension/supination/pronation are performed to reestablish proprioception and neuromuscular control.

Phase 2: Intermediate

Phase 2, the intermediate phase, is initiated when the following are achieved: full throwing ROM (as it was prior to the injury), minimal pain and tenderness, and a good (≥ 4/5) manual muscle test of the elbow flexor and extensor musculature. The emphasis of this phase includes maintaining and enhancing elbow and upper extremity mobility, improving muscular strength and endurance, and re-establishing neuromuscular control of the elbow complex.

Stretching exercises are continued to maintain full elbow and wrist ROM. Mobilization techniques may be progressed to more aggressive grade III and IV techniques as needed to apply a stretch to the capsular tissue at end range. Flexibility is progressed during this phase to focus on wrist flexion, extension, pronation, and supination. Elbow extension and forearm pronation flexibility are of particular emphasis in throwing athletes to perform efficiently. Shoulder flexibility is also maintained with emphasis on external and internal rotation at 90° of abduction, flexion, and horizontal adduction. In particular, shoulder external rotation at 90° abduction is emphasized; loss of external rotation may result in increased strain on the medial elbow structures during the overhead throwing motion. Additionally, internal rotation motion is also diligently performed, as internal rotation range of motion of the shoulder may create a protective varus force at the elbow. The rehabilitation program for shoulder joint ROM should consider the total ROM, and appropriate treatments should be employed to restore equal motion bilaterally.

Strengthening exercises are progressed during this phase to include isotonic contractions, beginning with concentric and progressing to include eccentric. Emphasis is placed on elbow flexion and extension, wrist flexion and extension, and forearm pronation and supination. The glenohumeral and scapulothoracic muscles are also placed on a progressive resistance program if there is no elbow pain. Emphasis is placed on strengthening the shoulder external rotators and periscapular muscles. A complete upper extremity strengthening program, such as the Thrower's Ten program, may be performed. This program has been designed based on electromyographic studies to illicit activity of the muscles most needed to provide dynamic stability. Strengthening exercises are advanced to include external and internal rotation with exercise tubing at 0° of abduction and active ROM exercises against gravity. These exercises initially include standing scaption in external rotation (full can), standing abduction, side-lying external rotation, and prone rowing. As strength returns, the program may be advanced to full upper extremity strengthening with emphasis on posterior rotator cuff muscles and scapular strengthening. Recently, a 6-week training program utilizing the Thrower's Ten program resulted in a 2-mph increase in throwing velocity in high school baseball pitchers.

Neuromuscular control exercises are initiated in this phase to enhance the muscles' ability to control the elbow joint during athletic activities. A decrease in neuromuscular control has also been associated with muscular fatigue. Detection of both internal and external rotation decreases following isokinetic fatigue protocol A significant decrease in accuracy occurs following muscle fatigue during both active and passive joint reproduction. Fatigue of the shoulder rotators results in decreased accuracy at mid- and end ROM. These exercises include proprioceptive neuromuscular facilitation with rhythmic stabilizations and manual resistance elbow/wrist flexion drills.

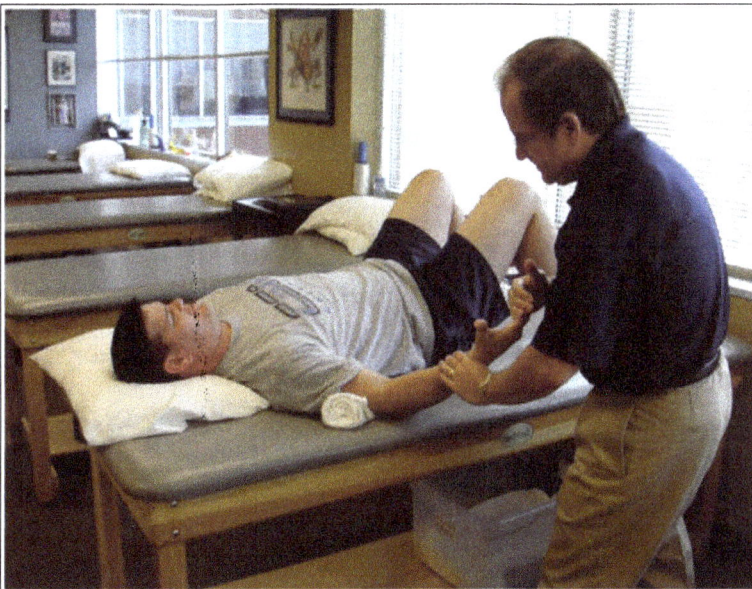

Manual concentric and eccentric resistance exercises for the
elbow flexors and wrist flexor-pronators.

Phase 3: Advanced Strengthening

The third phase involves a progression of activities to prepare the athlete for sport participation. The goals of this phase are to gradually increase strength, power, endurance, and neuromuscular control to prepare for a gradual return to sport. Specific criteria that must be met before entering this phase include full nonpainful external and internal rotation total ROM, no pain or tenderness, and strength that is 70% of the contralateral extremity.

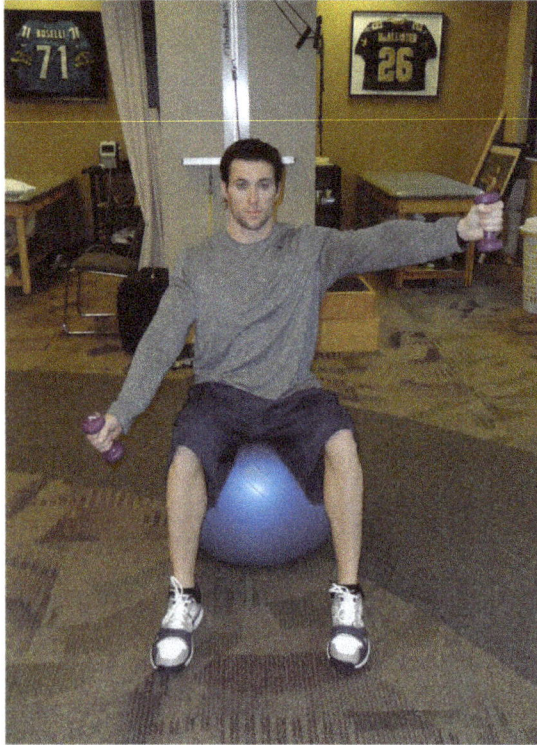

Advanced Thrower's Ten: Full can raises with sustained holds while seated on a stability ball.

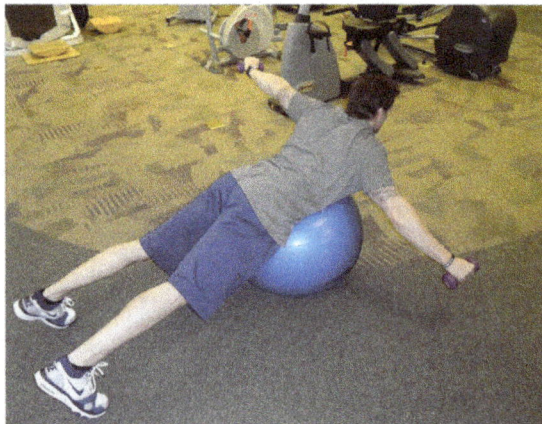

Advanced Thrower's Ten: Prone horizontal abduction on a stability ball while performing sustained holds.

Advanced strengthening activities during this phase include a gradual progression to higher resistance, functional movements, eccentric contraction, and plyometric activities. Elbow flexion exercises are progressed to emphasize eccentric control. The biceps muscle is an important stabilizer during the follow-through phase of overhead throwing. Eccentric control decelerates the elbow, preventing pathological abutting of the olecranon within the fossa. Elbow flexion can be performed with elastic tubing to emphasize slow- and fast-speed concentric and eccentric contractions. Furthermore, manual resistance may be applied for concentric and eccentric contractions of the elbow flexors. Aggressive strengthening exercises with weight machines are also incorporated during this phase when the athlete demonstrates the use of machines with an appropriate weight. These most commonly begin with bench press, seated rowing, and front latissimus dorsi pull-downs. The triceps are primarily exercised with a concentric contraction due to the muscle-shortening activity during the acceleration phase of throwing. During this phase, the overhead athlete may be placed on the Advanced Thrower's Ten program. This program incorporates exercises and movement patterns specific to the throwing motion, in a discrete series, utilizing principles of coactivation, high-level neuromuscular control, dynamic stabilization, muscular facilitation, endurance, and coordination that restore muscle balance and symmetry in the throwing athlete. Examples include the full can raise with sustained holds while seated on a stability ball or prone horizontal abduction on a stability ball while performing sustained holds.

Neuromuscular control exercises are progressed to side-lying external rotation with manual resistance. Concentric and eccentric external rotation is performed against the clinician's resistance with the addition of rhythmic stabilizations at end range. This manual resistance exercise may be progressed to external rotation with exercise tubing at 0° while seated on a physioball and finally at 90°of abduction.

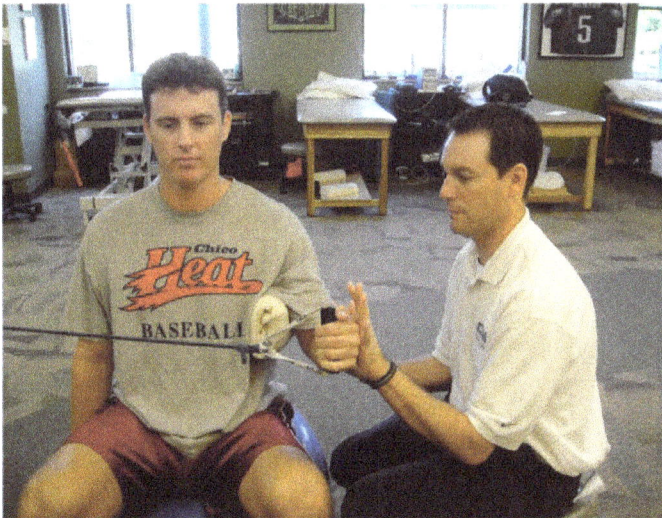

External rotation at 0° abduction with exercise tubing, manual resistance, and rhythmic stabilizations while the athlete is seated on a stability ball.

Plyometric drills can be an extremely beneficial functional exercise for training the elbow in overhead athletes. Plyometric exercises are performed using a weighted medicine ball during the later stages of this phase to train the shoulder and elbow to withstand high levels of stress. Plyometric exercises are initially performed with 2 hands (chest pass, side-to-side throw, and overhead soccer throw). These may be progressed to one-handed activities such as 90/90 throws with rhythmic stabilization at end range, external and internal rotation throws at 0° of abduction into a trampoline, and wall dribbles to improve shoulder endurance. Specific plyometric drills for the forearm musculature include wrist flexion flips and extension grips. The latter 2 plyometric drills are an important component of an elbow rehabilitation program, emphasizing the forearm and hand musculature. Plyometric training increases throwing velocity in high school baseball players.

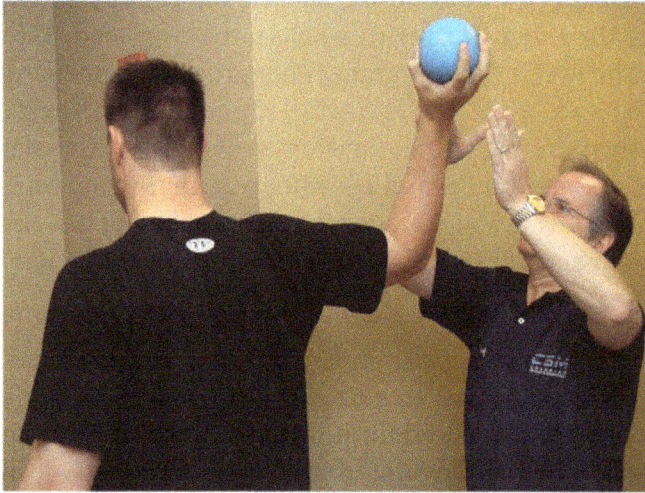

Plyometric wall throws with a 2-lb (0.91 kg) ball while the rehabilitation specialist performs a rhythmic stabilization at end range.

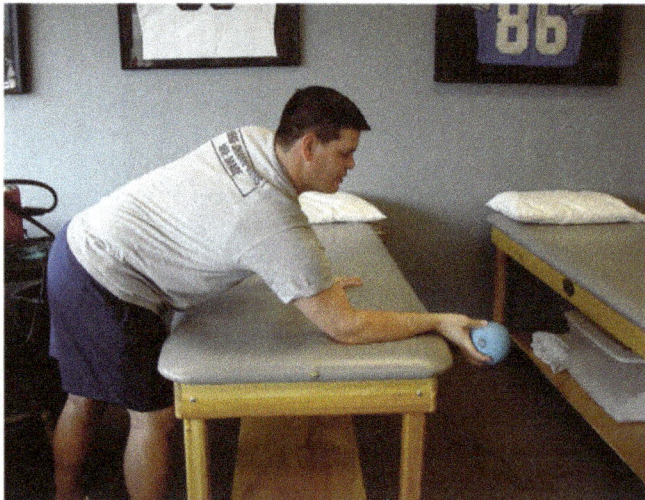

Plyometric wrist flips using a 2-lb (0.91 kg) medicine ball to strengthen the wrist flexors.

Phase 4: Return to Activity

The final phase of elbow rehabilitation, return to activity, allows the athlete to progressively return to full competition using an interval throwing program. Interval programs are used for the tennis player and golfer.

Before an athlete is allowed to begin the return-to-activity phase, he or she must exhibit full pain-free throwing ROM, no pain or tenderness, a satisfactory isokinetic test, and medical clearance through MD clinical examination. Isokinetic testing is commonly utilized to determine the readiness of the athlete to begin an interval sport program. Athletes are routinely tested at 180 and 300 degrees per second. Data indicate the bilateral comparison at 180 degrees per second for the throwing arm's elbow flexion 10% to 20% stronger and the dominant extensors, typically 5% to 15% stronger. Also, the athlete's ability to perform sport-specific drills with a Plyoball is evaluated. These drills include one-hand Plyoball wall throws stabilization and throwing into rebounder (1-lb [0.45 kg] Plyoball) from 20 ft (6.10 m). Each one of these drills is evaluated for pain, technique, and quality of movement.

Upon the achievement of the previous goals, a formal interval sport program can begin. For sports that involve the upper extremity, such as golf, tennis, baseball, and softball, an interval sport program is used. For the overhead thrower, we initiate a long-toss interval throwing program beginning at 45 ft (13.72 m) and gradually progressing to 120 or 180 feet (36.58 or 54.86 m; player and position dependent). Throwing should be performed without pain or significant increase in symptoms. During the long-toss program, as intensity and distance increase, the stresses increase on the patient's medial elbow and anterior shoulder joint. The longer throwing distances significantly increased these forces. It is important for the overhead athlete to perform stretching and an abbreviated strengthening program prior to and after performing the interval sport program. Typically, overhead throwers warm up, stretch, and perform 1 set of their exercise program before throwing, followed by 2 additional sets of exercises proceeding throwing. This provides an adequate warm-up but also ensures maintenance of necessary ROM and flexibility of the shoulder joint. The following day, the thrower will exercise his or her scapular muscles, external rotators, and perform a core stabilization program.

Following the completion of a long-toss program, pitchers will progress to phase II, throwing off a mound (Supplemental Table 4b). In phase II, the number of throws, intensity, and type of pitch are progressed to gradually increase stress on the elbow and shoulder joints. Generally, the pitcher begins at 50% intensity and gradually progresses to 75%, 90%, and 100% over a 4- to 6-week period. Breaking balls are initiated once the pitcher can throw 40 to 50 pitches at a minimum of 80% intensity without symptoms.

Specific Nonoperative Rehabilitation Guidelines

UCL Injury

Injuries to the UCL are becoming increasingly more common in overhead throwing athletes, although the higher incidence of injury may be due to the ability to detect these injuries. The elbow experiences a tremendous valgus stress during overhead throwing. The repetitive nature of overhead throwing activities further increases the susceptibility of UCL injury by exposing the ligament to repetitive microtraumatic forces.

Conservative treatment is attempted with partial tears and sprains of the UCL, although surgical reconstruction may be warranted for complete tears or if nonoperative treatment is unsuccessful. In the nonoperative rehabilitation program, ROM is initially permitted in a nonpainful arc of motion, usually from 10° to 100°, to decrease inflammation and align collagen tissue. A brace may be used to restrict motion and prevent valgus loading. Furthermore, it may be beneficial to rest the UCL immediately following the initial painful episode to prevent additional deleterious stress on the ligament. Isometric exercises are performed for the shoulder, elbow, and wrist to prevent muscular atrophy. Ice and anti-inflammatory medications are prescribed to control pain and inflammation.

ROM of flexion and extension is gradually increased by 5° to 10° per week during the second phase of treatment or as tolerated. Full pain-free ROM should be achieved by 3 to 4 weeks. Elbow flexion/extension motion is encouraged to promote collagen formation and alignment. Valgus loading of the elbow joint is controlled to minimize stress on the UCL. Rhythmic stabilization exercises are initiated to develop dynamic stabilization and neuromuscular control of the upper extremity. As dynamic stability is advanced, isotonic exercises are incorporated for the entire upper extremity.

The advanced strengthening phase is usually initiated at 6 to 7 weeks postinjury. During this phase, the athlete is progressed to the Thrower's Ten isotonic strengthening program, and plyometric exercises are slowly initiated. An interval return to throwing is initiated once the athlete regains full motion, adequate shoulder and elbow strength (5/5 manual muscle test), and dynamic stability of the elbow. The athlete is allowed to return to competition following the asymptomatic completion of the interval sport program. If symptoms reoccur during the interval throwing program, it is usually at longer distances, at greater intensities, or with off-the-mound throwing. If symptoms continue to persist, surgical intervention is considered.

Medial Epicondylitis and Flexor-Pronator Tendinitis

Medial epicondylitis pain occurs within the flexor-pronator musculotendinous unit. Nirschl et al reported 4 stages of epicondylitis, beginning with an early inflammatory reaction, followed by angiofibroblastic degeneration, leading to structural failure, and ultimately, fibrosis or calcification. It is critical to identify the condition of the tendon because the stage of the injury will dictate treatment.

The treatment for tendonitis is typically targeted at reducing inflammation and pain through a reduction in activities, steroid injections, anti-inflammatory medications, cryotherapy, iontophoresis, light exercise, and stretching.

The nonoperative approach for treatment of epicondylitis (ie, tendinitis and/or para-tendinitis) focuses on pain and inflammation control and then gradual improvement in muscular strength. The initial treatment consists of modalities, stretching exercises, and light strengthening to stimulate a repair response. Common modalities include massage, cold laser therapy, iontophoresis (Hybresis DJO Global, Vista, California), ultrasound, nitric oxide, and extracorporeal shockwave therapy. When these are used in combination with exercise or with other modalities, improved tissue quality and outcomes may be realized.

Once the patient's symptoms have subsided, an aggressive stretching and (high-load, low-repetitions) strengthening program with emphasis on eccentric contractions is initiated. Wrist flexion and extension activities should be performed initially with the elbow flexed 30° to 45° to decrease stress on the medial elbow structures. A gradual progression through plyometric and throwing activities precedes initiating the interval throwing program.

Conversely, the treatment for tendinosis focuses on increasing circulation to promote collagen synthesis and collagen organization. Heat, stretching, eccentrics, laser therapy, transverse massage, and soft tissue mobilization are utilized to increase circulation and promote tissue healing. Dry needling may promote tendon healing. Eccentric exercise and strength training can improve results by increasing collagen synthesis and improving fiber orientation. Laser therapy and extracorporeal shockwave therapy have also shown promising results.

The goal of these treatments is to stimulate a regenerative response that otherwise would not occur. Platelet-rich plasma (PRP) is promising by delivering humoral mediators and growth factors locally to induce a healing response. Mishra et al showed significant benefits to PRP in chronic lateral epicondylitis. Thanasas et al showed improved visual analog scale scores in ultrasound-guided PRP injections. In a randomized controlled double-blind study, improved visual analog scale scores and DASH (Disabilities of the Arm, Shoulder and Hand) scores were seen in the PRP group compared with a corticosteroid group even at a 2-year follow-up in patients with chronic lateral epicondylitis. Basic science and controlled studies have yet to truly surmise the efficacy of PRP.

Valgus Extension Overload

Valgus extension overload occurs during repetitive, forceful extension: during the acceleration or deceleration phase of throwing as the olecranon wedges up against the medial olecranon. This may result in osteophyte formation and potentially loose bodies. Repetitive extension stress from the triceps may further contribute to this injury. There is often underlying valgus laxity of the elbow, further facilitating osteophyte formation through compression of the radiocapitellar joint and the posteromedial elbow. Overhead athletes typically present with pain at the posteromedial elbow that is exacerbated with forced extension and valgus stress.

A conservative initial treatment involves relieving pain and inflammation with ice, laser, and iontophoresis. As symptoms subside and ROM normalizes, dynamic stabilization and strengthening exercises are initiated with emphasis on eccentric strength of the elbow flexors to control rapid extension at the elbow. Manual resistance exercises of concentric and eccentric elbow flexion are performed, as well as elbow flexion with exercise tubing. The athlete's throwing mechanics should be carefully assessed to determine if mechanical faults are causing the valgus extension overload symptoms or if a UCL injury is present.

Osteochondritis Dissecans

Osteochondritis dissecans of the elbow may develop because of the valgus strain on the elbow joint, which produces not only medial tension but also a lateral compressive force as the capitellum compresses the radial head. Patients often complain of lateral elbow pain upon palpation and valgus stress. Morrey described a 3-stage classification of pathological progression: stage 1, no evidence of subchondral displacement or fracture; stage 2, evidence of subchondral detachment or articular cartilage fracture; stage 3, detached osteochondral fragments, resulting intra-articular loose bodies. Nonsurgical treatment is attempted for stage 1 patients, only consisting of relative rest and immobilization until elbow symptoms.

Nonoperative treatment includes 3 to 6 weeks of immobilization at 90° of elbow flexion. ROM activities for the shoulder, elbow, and wrist are performed 3 to 4 times a day. As symptoms resolve, a strengthening program is initiated with isometric exercises. Isotonic exercises are included after approximately 1 week of isometric exercise. Aggressive high-speed, eccentric, and plyometric exercises are progressively included to prepare the athlete for the start of an interval throwing program.

If nonoperative treatment fails or evidence of loose bodies exists, surgical intervention is indicated, including arthroscopic abrading and drilling of the lesion with fixation or removal of the loose body. Long-term follow-up studies regarding the outcome of patients undergoing surgery to drill or reattach the lesions have not produced favorable results suggesting that prevention and early detection of symptoms may be the best form of treatment.

Little League Elbow

Little League elbow is a spectrum of medial epicondylar apophyseal injury that ranges from microtrauma to the physis to fracture and displacement of the medial epicondyle through the apophysis. Pain of the medial elbow is common in adolescent throwers. The medial epicondyle physis is subject to repetitive tensile and valgus forces during the arm-cocking and acceleration phases of throwing. These forces may result in micro-traumatic injury to the physis with potential fragmentation, hypertrophy, separation of the epiphysis, or avulsion of the medial epicondyle. Treatment varies based on the extent of injury.

In the absence of an avulsion, a rehabilitation program similar to that of the nonop-erative UCL program is initiated. Emphasis is placed on the reduction of pain and inflammation and the restoration of motion and strength. Strengthening exercises are performed in a gradual fashion; isometrics are prior to light isotonic exercises. In young throwing athletes, core, legs, and shoulder strengthening is encouraged. Often, these individuals exhibit poor core and scapula control along with weakness of the shoulder musculature. In addition, stretching exercises are performed to nor-malize shoulder ROM, especially into internal rotation and horizontal adduction. No heavy lifting is permitted for 12 to 14 weeks. An interval throwing program is initiated as tolerated when symptoms subside, typically after an 8- to 12-week rest period.

In the presence of a non-displaced or minimally displaced avulsion, a brief period of immobilization for approximately 7 to 14 days is encouraged, followed by a gradual progression of ROM, flexibility, and strength. An interval throwing program is usually allowed at weeks 8 to 12. If the avulsion is displaced, an open-reduction, internal-fixa-tion procedure may be required.

Specific Postoperative Rehabilitation Guidelines

UCL Reconstruction

Surgical reconstruction of the UCL attempts to restore the stabilizing functions of the anterior bundle of the UCL. Several surgical procedures exist, including the Jobe pro-cedure, the docking procedure, and the DANE procedure. The modified Jobe procedure uses the palmaris longus or gracilis graft in a figure pattern through drill holes in the sublime tubercle of the ulna and the medial epicondyle. A subcutaneous ulnar nerve transposition is performed at the time of reconstruction.

The rehabilitation program following UCL reconstruction is based on the surgical pro-cedure. The athlete is in a posterior splint with the elbow immobilized at 90° of flexion for the first 7 days postoperatively. This allows early healing of the UCL graft and fas-cial slings involved in the nerve transposition. Wrist ROM gripping and submaximal isometrics for the wrist and elbow are allowed. The patient is progressed from the pos-terior splint to a hinged elbow ROM brace to protect the healing tissues from valgus stresses after 4 weeks.

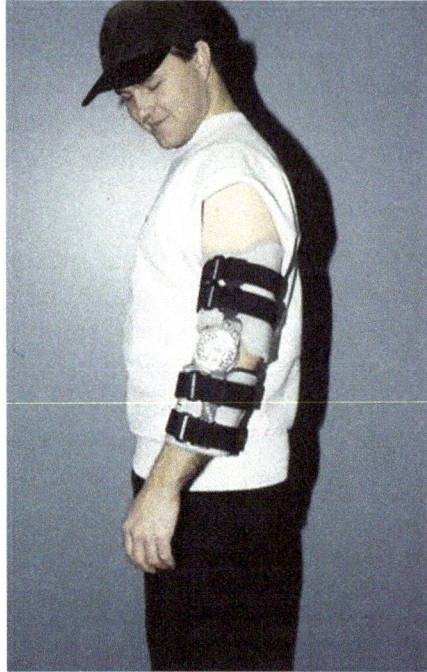

Hinged elbow brace utilized postoperatively to protect
the graft from deleterious valgus stresses.

Passive ROM activities are initiated immediately to decrease pain and slowly stress the healing tissues. Initially, the focus of the rehabilitation is obtaining full elbow extension while gradually progressing flexion. Elbow extension is encouraged early on to at least 15°, but if the patient can comfortably obtain full extension, then it is allowed as long as there is no discomfort. Passive ROM of the elbow joint produces 3% strain or less in both bands of the reconstructed ligament and approximately 1% strain for the anterior band of the UCL. In the immediate postoperative period, full elbow extension is safe and does not place excessive stress on the healing graft. Conversely, elbow flexion to 100° is allowed and increased 10° per week until full ROM is achieved by 4 to 6 weeks postoperatively.

Isometric exercises are progressed to include light resistance isotonic exercises at weeks 3 to 4, while the Thrower's Ten program is initiated by week 6. Progressive resistance exercises are incorporated at weeks 8 to 9. Focus is placed on developing dynamic stabilization of the medial elbow. Because of the anatomic orientation of the flexor carpi ulnaris and flexor digitorum superficialis overlaying the UCL, isotonic and stabilization activities may assist the UCL in stabilizing valgus stress at the medial elbow.

Aggressive exercises involving eccentric and plyometric contractions are in the advanced phase (weeks 12-16), while the advanced Thrower's Ten program is initiated at week 12. Two-hand plyometric drills are performed at week 12, one-hand drills at week 14, and an interval throwing program at week 16 postoperatively. In most cases, throwing from a mound occurs 4 to 6 weeks following the initiation of interval throwing, and a return to competitive throwing, at approximately 9 months following surgery.

UCL reconstruction in 743 athletes during a 2-year minimum follow-up with subcutaneous ulnar nerve transposition was effective in correcting valgus elbow instability in the overhead athlete and allowed most athletes (83%) to return to previous or higher levels of competition in less than 1 year. Major complications were noted in 4% of the athletes.

The rehabilitation program following UCL reconstruction utilizing the docking procedure is slightly different. An elbow brace with ROM from 30° to 60° is used for the first 3 weeks; 15° to 90° at week 4. The athlete should obtain full ROM by 6 weeks. Isotonic strengthening exercises are initiated at week 6. Plyometric activities may be performed at approximately 10 weeks to further stress the healing tissues in preparation for the interval throwing program. The athlete may incorporate heavier strengthening exercises utilizing machine weights at this time. A positional player may begin a hitting program at 12 weeks: first hitting off of a tee, progressing to soft-toss throws and, finally, formal batting practice. The interval throwing program is permitted at 4 months postoperatively, and formal pitching is typically accomplished at 9 months.

Ulnar Nerve Transposition

Ulnar nerve transposition is often performed in a subcutaneous fashion using fascial slings. Caution is taken to avoid stressing the soft tissue surrounding the nerve while healing occurs. A posterior splint at 90° of elbow flexion is used for the first week to prevent excessive flexion and tension on the nerve. The splint is discharged at week 2, and light ROM activities are initiated. Full ROM is usually restored by weeks 3 to 4. Gentle isotonic strengthening is begun during weeks 3 to 4 and progressed to the full Thrower's Ten program by 4 to 6 weeks. Aggressive strengthening, including eccentric, advanced Thrower's Ten, and plyometric training, is incorporated at week 8, and an interval throwing program, at weeks 10 to 12, if all criteria are met, similar to the advanced phase of the UCL protocol. A return to competition usually occurs at week 16 postoperatively.

Posterior Olecranon Osteophyte Excision

The rehabilitation program following arthroscopic posterior olecranon osteophyte excision is slightly more conservative in restoring full elbow extension secondary to postsurgical pain. ROM is progressed within the patient's tolerance; by 10 days postoperative, the patient should exhibit at least 15 to 105/110 degrees of ROM, and 5-10 to 115° by day 14. Full ROM (0°-145°) is typically restored by days 20 to 25. The rate of ROM progression is most often limited by osseous pain and synovial joint inflammation, usually located at the tip of the olecranon.

Isometrics are performed for the first 10 to 14 days, and isotonic strengthening, from weeks 2 to 6. Initially, especially during the first 2 weeks, forceful triceps contractions may produce posterior elbow pain. If present, the force produced by the triceps muscle should be avoided or reduced. The full Thrower's Ten program is initiated by week 6, with interval throwing program by weeks 10 to 12. The rehabilitation focus is similar to the nonoperative treatment of valgus extension overload with emphasis on eccentric control of the elbow flexors and dynamic stabilization of the medial elbow.

In 72 professional baseball players undergoing elbow surgery, 65% exhibited a posterior olecranon osteophyte. Twenty-five percent later required an UCL reconstruction, suggesting that subtle medial instability may accelerate osteophyte formation.

The elbow joint is a common site of injury in the overhead athlete due to the repetitive microtraumatic injuries. In collision sports, elbow injury is often due to macrotraumatic forces resulting in fractures, dislocations, and ligamentous injuries. Rehabilitation of the elbow, whether postinjury or postsurgical, must be progressive and sequential to ensure that healing tissues are not overstressed but provide appropriate stress to promote proper collagen alignment. The rehabilitation program should limit immobilization and achieve full ROM early, especially elbow extension. The rehabilitation program must progressively restore strength and neuromuscular control while gradually incorporating sports-specific activities to successfully return the athlete to his or her previous level of function as quickly and safely as possible. The rehabilitation of the elbow must include the entire kinetic chain (scapula, shoulder, hand, core/hips, and legs) to ensure the athlete's return to high-level sports participation.

References

- Rehabilitation-in-Sport: physio-pedia.com, Retrieved 16 April, 2019

- What-is-sports-specific-rehabilitation: truesportsphysicaltherapy.com, Retrieved 18 July, 2019

- Sports-concussion: now.aapmr.org, Retrieved 19 June, 2019

- Sports-and-occupational-injuries-to-the-wrist-and-hand: now.aapmr.org, Retrieved 15 March, 2019

- Shin-splints: physio-pedia.com, Retrieved 07 January, 2019

Permissions

All chapters in this book are published with permission under the Creative Commons Attribution Share Alike License or equivalent. Every chapter published in this book has been scrutinized by our experts. Their significance has been extensively debated. The topics covered herein carry significant information for a comprehensive understanding. They may even be implemented as practical applications or may be referred to as a beginning point for further studies.

We would like to thank the editorial team for lending their expertise to make the book truly unique. They have played a crucial role in the development of this book. Without their invaluable contributions this book wouldn't have been possible. They have made vital efforts to compile up to date information on the varied aspects of this subject to make this book a valuable addition to the collection of many professionals and students.

This book was conceptualized with the vision of imparting up-to-date and integrated information in this field. To ensure the same, a matchless editorial board was set up. Every individual on the board went through rigorous rounds of assessment to prove their worth. After which they invested a large part of their time researching and compiling the most relevant data for our readers.

The editorial board has been involved in producing this book since its inception. They have spent rigorous hours researching and exploring the diverse topics which have resulted in the successful publishing of this book. They have passed on their knowledge of decades through this book. To expedite this challenging task, the publisher supported the team at every step. A small team of assistant editors was also appointed to further simplify the editing procedure and attain best results for the readers.

Apart from the editorial board, the designing team has also invested a significant amount of their time in understanding the subject and creating the most relevant covers. They scrutinized every image to scout for the most suitable representation of the subject and create an appropriate cover for the book.

The publishing team has been an ardent support to the editorial, designing and production team. Their endless efforts to recruit the best for this project, has resulted in the accomplishment of this book. They are a veteran in the field of academics and their pool of knowledge is as vast as their experience in printing. Their expertise and guidance has proved useful at every step. Their uncompromising quality standards have made this book an exceptional effort. Their encouragement from time to time has been an inspiration for everyone.

The publisher and the editorial board hope that this book will prove to be a valuable piece of knowledge for students, practitioners and scholars across the globe.

Index

A

Ai Chi, 27

Amyotrophic Lateral Sclerosis, 22, 42, 60, 71, 75, 85

Ankle Sprains, 11, 195, 199-200

Anxiety, 51, 177, 206, 208-209

Aqua Running, 27

Aquatic Therapy, 20, 23-24, 26-31, 103, 126

Arthritis, 4-5, 12, 19, 21, 24-26, 28, 82, 125, 139, 156, 160, 172, 174, 204, 214-217, 219

Arthrogryposis, 43, 54, 139

Autism, 25

B

Becker Muscular Dystrophy, 43-44, 72, 112

Biomechanical Movements, 1

Bone Structures, 11

Burdenko Method, 28

Bursitis, 18, 25, 147, 151-152, 161, 170-172

C

Calcific Tendonitis, 5, 150, 159

Cardiac Event, 35-37

Cardiac Rehabilitation, 35-37

Cardiovascular Endurance, 23, 185

Cardiovascular System, 36, 39, 98, 184

Central Nervous System, 22, 44, 77, 79, 107, 128, 141

Cerebral Palsy, 4, 11, 25, 38, 105-108, 110-111, 126, 136, 138

Charlevoix Regions, 44, 50

Chest Physical Therapy, 14

Clapping, 14-15, 94

Cognitive Rehabilitation Therapy, 14, 32, 35

Corpus Callosum, 50

Cystic Fibrosis, 14

D

Deep Vein Thrombosis, 6, 223

Desmin Myopathy, 52

Diabetes Mellitus, 49, 155

Dysphagia, 58, 71, 74

E

Enzyme Replacement Therapy, 59

F

Fractured Femur, 2

Functional Training, 38, 141, 190

G

Genetic Mutation, 42

Geriatric Physical Therapy, 14, 19-21

H

Halliwick Concept, 28

Heat Treatments, 5

Hip Fracture, 19

Hydrotherapy, 23, 28-29, 106, 166, 196

I

Intensive Care Unit, 36, 46, 133

L

Ligament Sprains, 18, 171, 187

Lokomat, 38

M

Malformation, 1, 132

Manual Muscle Testing, 62-63, 84, 98

Manual Therapy, 13, 20, 39, 118, 145, 165-167, 228

Maximal Expiratory Pressure, 68

Mitochondria, 49, 53

Motor Function Measure, 67, 140

Movement Therapy, 1, 107

Multicore Myopathy, 54

Muscle Strains, 17, 187

Muscle Strength, 11, 20, 24, 51, 62, 64, 66, 68, 72, 74, 77-79, 81, 83-84, 86, 89-92, 94, 96, 109-110

Musculoskeletal Medicine, 12-13

Myasthenia Gravis, 43, 55, 60, 71, 75, 105

Myositis Disorders, 55

N

Nemaline Myopathy, 57, 75

Nerve Biopsy, 10

Neuromuscular Function, 2, 189, 192

Neuromuscular Medicine, 41, 60-61

O

Occupational Therapists, 23, 33, 117, 125-126, 136, 140, 142, 210

Orthopedic Physical Therapy, 14, 17-18

Osteoporosis, 4, 9, 19, 119, 170-172

P

Parkinson's Disease, 21-22, 25, 28, 144, 176-177

Perceived Exertion, 37

Peripheral Nervous System, 42, 44, 71, 79, 104, 127, 129

Physical Medicine, 1-2, 9, 24, 61, 144, 179

Physical Therapy, 2, 4-5, 7, 14, 17-23, 43, 59, 97, 99, 103, 106, 114, 116, 126, 143, 158, 160-161, 167-168, 170-171, 174, 177, 181, 193, 226, 228

Physiotherapy, 10-13, 51-52, 89, 94, 105, 135, 143, 190

Pompe Disease, 58

Postural Drainage, 14

Pulmonary Embolism, 6

R

Rehabilitation Medicine, 9-10, 14, 104, 125, 136, 183

Respiratory Care, 46-47

Robotic Neurorehabilitation, 14, 37-38

S

Sepsis, 8

Side Shuffling, 31

Spinal Cord, 4, 9, 13, 22, 25, 38, 41, 43-44, 49, 60, 71, 104, 128, 132, 134, 136, 139, 144, 159

Spinal Muscular Atrophy, 42, 59, 71, 73

Steroid Injections, 5, 239

T

Therapy Pool, 26, 30-32

Total Knee Replacement, 7

Traumatic Brain Injury, 22, 25, 38, 139

U

Underwater Treadmill, 27, 30

V

Visual Perceptual Skill, 23

www.ingramcontent.com/pod-product-compliance
Lightning Source LLC
Chambersburg PA
CBHW061936190326
41458CB00009B/2756